Practical Concepts and Training Exercises for Crisis Intervention Teams

Including Role-Plays and Interactive Games

Second Edition

Dennis Potter, MSW, CSW, FAAETS
James A. Stevens, MA
Paul LaBerteaux, PsyD

CHEVRON
PUBLISHING CORPORATION

COVER PHOTO:
Roger Hill, Photosphere Studios, Grand Rapids, Michigan

Printed in the United States of America

ISBN-13: 978-1-883581-34-3
ISBN-10: 1-883581-34-6

SECOND EDITION

CHEVRON
PUBLISHING CORPORATION
5018 Dorsey Hall Drive, Suite 104
Ellicott City, MD 21042
410-740-0065

Foreword

By Kendall Johnson, PhD

Crisis is no stranger to our communities, our workplaces, or to our schools. Anywhere people gather there is drama. Homes burn, autos crash, and parents die. In my work within schools, teachers, school psychologists, counselors, college deans, and coaches have always provided informal student support during emergencies. Gradually over the past 30 years, this support system has become formalized. Crisis intervention, specialized training in emergency mental health, and student support teams have become the order of the day.

Since the early 1980s when writings about Critical Incident Stress Management (CISM) first began to appear, the focus was always on first responders. Times have changed, however, and they present unprecedented challenges to communities and schools which require a broader, more comprehensive approach than ever before. The basics of individual crisis intervention are not enough to prepare schools adequately to meet student and staff needs following natural disasters, large-scale incidents, and civil unrest. Targeted school violence, bombs, and the growing specter of terrorist strikes on or near schools call for more flexible and thorough approaches to crisis response and management. Schools have never existed apart from their communities, but community events now reach the school more frequently and with greater intensity.

Training personnel to respond to emergencies takes special resources and this book provides just that. Dennis Potter, James Stevens, and Paul LaBerteaux bring years of hands-on crisis response experience to the table. I have known Dennis and Paul for years through my work with the International Critical Incident Stress Foundation. They work within the framework of Critical Incident Stress Management (Everly and Mitchell, 1999), a comprehensive, multi-component approach that addresses crisis issues from pre-incident preparation through post-incident follow-up and referral. This book utilizes CISM in a friendly, practical, no-nonsense manner that has important implications.

The first implication recognizes the growing trend toward multi-agency community and school crisis teams (Johnson, 2000; Tortorici Luna, 2002). This book encourages and employs a community-based and multi-agency approach. The authors recognize two critical aspects of contemporary crisis management. The first is that CISM teams can expect larger crises that involve the community. The second is that the community can provide precious human resources for the school. Coordination with community resources is critical, and school personnel working alone simply cannot provide the high standards of student care that communities expect.

With that comes the need to articulate a common language and shared strategies. In addition, school and community resources must work together in planning sessions to define the manner in which emergency responders and school personnel can coordinate their efforts to each other's benefit. Pre-incident planning provides this opportunity, and training provides the vehicle.

One of the strengths of this book is the compilation of simulation training scenarios. A number of interesting situations are provided for team exercises; these are carefully thought out and are field-tested. I was fortunate to teach for a time at the California Specialized Training Institute (training arm of the Office of Emergency Service and prototype for the FEMA Emergency Management Institute). CSTI has always utilized simulation exercises to assist emergency personnel in synthesizing diverse information and strategies and has become familiar with their orchestration. Learning is only partial until it results in action.

Productive simulations must move beyond rote role play. They must incorporate complex situations with variable options, unanticipated developments, and elements of duress to maximize training potential. I have tried to introduce such elements into my own team training.

This book is the first resource I have seen that provides a wealth of suggestions, scenarios, and situations appropriate for action-based team training. Simulation exercises are provided for fire/EMS, law enforcement, community, and school-based incidents, using multi-agency, multi-disciplinary crisis teams.

Finally, it must be recognized that community organizations and schools are not emergency agencies. If materials and approaches are to be useful and helpful within these settings, they must allow for flexible adaptation to meet the complex and multi-dimensional demands of the organization, culture, scope—and yes, political realities. The concepts and training exercises herein are highly practical. While they are firmly based upon solid theoretical ground, they are not dogmatic. The training approach utilized is suggestive and does not attempt to superimpose a rigid paramilitary structure. I am sure you will find ***Practical Concepts and Training Exercises For Crisis Intervention Teams*** both school- and community-friendly.

Potter, Stevens, and LaBerteaux are to be congratulated for providing a major and significant contribution to an essential field. Crisis management is becoming central to the safety of our nation, our community, and our children—and providing for the safety of our children is more necessary now than ever before.

References:

Everly, G., and Mitchell, J. 1999. *Critical Incident Stress Management (CISM): A New Era and Standard of Care in Crisis Intervention.* 2nd Ed. Ellicott City, MD: Chevron Publishing.

Johnson, K. 2000. *School Crisis Management: A Hands-on Guide to Training Crisis Response Teams,* 2nd Edition. Alameda, CA: Hunter House Publishers.

Tortorici Luna, J. 2002. "Adapting CISM to the schools: A multi-agency approach." Manuscript submitted for publication.

Acknowledgements

No book comes to print based solely upon the efforts of the authors. This guidebook is certainly no exception to this rule. The authors have been taught by Jeffery T. Mitchell and George Everly from the International Critical Incident Stress Foundation and their on-going efforts on behalf of those of us on the front lines.

We have also been enriched by our association with the members of the Michigan Crisis Response Association and the experience of having taught at their annual training conference over the years. Gregg Ginebaugh, Kathy Lewis, and Sue Elben have contributed their ideas to making the games more interesting and fun.

We have never conducted a training program in which we have not learned something from the participants. Of course, none of the training would be fruitful if it had not been put to use in providing CISM services. Our profound gratitude goes to those individuals participating in CISM activities over the years, which have taught us far more than any seminar.

During the development of this book, we have asked people to review and comment on our efforts and have been pleased that they have graciously done so. Kristin Gray, a member of the U.S. Coast Guard Pacific Northwest team and the WA CISM Network; Vaughn Donaldson of the Permian Basin CISM Team in Midland, TX; and Phyllis Hemmer, from Gryphon Place, in Kalamazoo, MI, have all contributed their comments and support for our efforts.

We owe a special tribute to Susan Potter, who faithfully pored over each draft offering comments and grammatical challenges. Dennis would also like to thank Susan for her unwavering support and encouragement during the writing of this guidebook.

Paul wishes to express his heartfelt appreciation to his love, Linda, not only for her support, but also for her technical tutoring and for her patience with him as he was "dragged kicking and screaming into the age of computers...or at least to its front door."

Thank you for your assistance in this effort and your support of our efforts over the years.

DMP
JAS
PL

Biography of the Authors

Dennis Potter, *MSW, CSW, BCSCR, BCETS, FAAETS*

Dennis Potter is a certified social worker, who along with Paul LaBerteaux, helped to form one of the first community-based crisis response teams in Michigan. Dennis was also one of the founding members of the Mid-West Michigan Critical Incident Stress Management (CISM) Team and the Michigan Crisis Response Association (MCRA). He is recognized as Board Certified School Crisis Response (BCSCR), an Expert in Traumatic Stress (BCETS), and a Fellow, the highest certification given, by the American Academy of Experts in Traumatic Stress.

Since 1989, Dennis has helped to train many of the CISM teams in Michigan and frequently is called upon for consultation after particularly difficult events. Through their association with these teams, Dennis and Paul have conducted or consulted on all manner of traumatic events for communities, businesses, schools, police, fire and emergency services personnel, the U.S. Post Office, and community mental health agencies.

Dennis has presented at many local, state, regional, national, and international conferences. He and Paul have been presenters at the International Critical Incident Stress Foundation World Congresses since 1995. Dennis has completed Trainers Training from ICISF and is certified as a Basic CISM, Advanced CISM, Individual Crisis Intervention and Peer Support, and CISM for Schools instructor. He has written articles for various journals on the topic of working with Critical Incident Stress. Dennis and Paul authored the model for *Debriefing the Debriefers* which is featured in the ICISF Advanced Training Workbook.

James Stevens, *MA*

Jim Stevens has BA and MA degrees in education and school administration and is a retired school administrator and teacher. He was a licensed paramedic in the State of Michigan for several years and retains his EMT (emergency medical technician) basic and his IC (instructor-coordinator) license. Jim is an adjunct faculty member with Kellogg Community College in Battle Creek, MI, where he teaches medical continuing education with area fire departments.

Jim received his ICISF training from Jeffrey Mitchell in 1992. He is a member of the Michigan Crisis Response Association Board of Directors and has served on the planning committee for the Annual MCRA Training Conference since 1996. At the MCRA Annual Conference, he has taught courses on Basic CISM for EMS, Level II CISM for EMS and Community Responders, and Difficult Debriefings. In addition, Jim has assisted Dennis Potter in teaching the Advanced CISM and is an ICISF certified instructor for CISM in the Schools.

Jim is the founding president of the Calhoun County, MI, CISM team and a coordinator for the Barry, Branch, and Calhoun County CISM teams.

***Paul LaBerteaux**, PsyD*

Paul LaBerteaux is a licensed clinical psychologist who, since 1975, has worked in community mental health and private practice. In 1990, Paul and Dennis formed a private consulting firm, Kantu Consultants, specializing in Critical Incident Stress Management. Paul's specialties have been community-based and school populations. Over the last 15 years, Paul has helped to train hundreds of crisis teams throughout Michigan, and has been especially focused on school-based teams in West Michigan.

Paul helped to form one of the country's first community-based CISM teams in 1985, and continues to serve as coordinator of this group of 60 trained volunteers after more than 400 responses. His training service through the Michigan Crisis Response Association at their yearly conference has helped to establish teams across the state. Paul has a wealth of practical experience and imparts it in a relaxed and effective manner, building skills through experience and practice. He has presented at many conferences at the local, state, national, and international level.

Paul and Dennis have been presenters at the International Critical Incident Stress Foundation World Congresses since 1995. Paul has completed Trainers Training from ICISF and is certified as a Basic CISM, Individual Crisis Intervention and Peer Support, and CISM for Schools instructor. Dennis and Paul authored the model for *Debriefing the Debriefers* which is featured in the ICISF Advanced Training Workbook.

Table of Contents

Introduction

This guidebook is designed to be used as a practical resource for team coordinators in developing and maintaining a Critical Incident Stress Management (CISM) team. It provides those responsible for the ongoing development and training of a team with ready-made exercises and games which promote learning in a safe environment. The target of this guidebook's exercises is practice of the following interventions: Individual (one-on-one), Defusing, Debriefing (CISD), and Crisis Management Briefing (CMB). With creativity, the material in the scripts could serve as the basis for practice of any of the other six CISM interventions, but the intent was to focus on the four interventions named.

The guidebook is divided into five sections:

Section 1 is an overview of the CISM field and is designed to help train others in various responses thus helping to "raise the bar" for delivering CISM services.

Section 2 contains tips on operational guidelines that have been found especially important to the maintenance of a CISM team.

Section 3 represents the authors' attempts to pass along their favorite secrets and techniques for training. Some are widely used and will be familiar. Others are original with the authors. They vary on a continuum from those which teach one building block at a time in a cognitive way, to those which involve practice of complex situations under some emotional pressure. The experiential area of this section includes descriptions and instructions for five techniques: table-top exercises, role plays, group problem exercises, training games, and a model for debriefing the CISM team.

Section 4 is comprised of dozens of practice scenarios for use in a variety of exercises, e.g., one-on-one, table-top, role plays, group briefings, etc. These scenarios are divided by population (firefighter/EMS, law enforcement, school, and community groups) and contain a wide range of topics and issues. Each scenario comes complete with an instruction sheet for six to nine participants, which describes their role in the incident and some suggestions for thoughts and reactions they might have.

Section 5 is a collection of group exercises and educational games, the more complex of which are included on PowerPoint on the accompanying CD. They are designed for use when time is short, provide skill practice of a lively nature, and are fun ways to end a meeting or training on a high note.

Finally, the **Appendix** contains a variety of forms and a suggested reading list which have been found useful in accomplishing some of the goals proposed in the text.

This book is not intended to replace the book, *Critical Incident Stress Debriefing: An Operations Manual for CISD, Defusing and Other Group Crisis Intervention Services* by Mitchell and Everly (2001), but rather as a companion book based upon its important precepts. All CISM responders should be familiar with this text.

Why Script a Scenario?

It is a basic truth that most people do not really like to participate in role plays. Anyone who uses them as a regular technique will tell you that it is difficult to get volunteers. But participant evaluations consistently bear out what the education texts teach—there is nothing like experiential learning. The evolution of training efforts in CISM reveals their increasing use by most instructors. The real question is not whether to use them, but how to use them.

It is quite possible to do a good role play on an impromptu basis, provided you have some willing participants. Simply describe an event, assign each participant some role in it, and let them use their imaginations. But scripting a role play, with written suggestions for each role, has some definite advantages. Since this is the primary rationale for much of this book, it seems appropriate to list some of those advantages here.

There are some issues which will seldom get presented spontaneously in an unscripted role play. Some issues are simply unusual or occur infrequently. Some issues are inherently threatening and will be avoided as much by role players as they are by our real-life debriefees. How many role players will make up details such as physical contact with damaged bodies, the expression on a dying victim's face, or tunnel vision? How many would give you valuable examples of irrational blaming, or anger directed at a dead colleague after a suicide? Scripting is one way to make sure the range of thoughts, reactions, and symptoms portrayed in a role play at least approximates real life. Scripting can allow the trainer to target specific lessons. Want your group to focus on ways to handle anger and blaming? Give them a script in which several characters are told to present those issues.

Believe it or not, most role plays end up being tougher than the average real life response. Role players have a tendency to present their own worst case scenario or worst fear. Also, role players often don't know each other as well as real life participants do and thus are not as spontaneously supportive of one another. Often, these factors combine to leave an unrealistically negative picture in the minds of new trainees. Scripting allows us to sprinkle groups with naturally helping characters, unaffected characters, and more realistic symptoms. Scripting a role play can bring out the good in groups, just like real life. Also, following the instructions labeled "Getting Started" and "Instructions to Participants" will help avoid the more common pitfalls of role play.

An innovation called the "Table-Top Exercise" is described. It uses the same scenarios, but provides for a less threatening, slow motion walk-through of the group process. It has shown itself to be especially helpful in building newer team members' understanding of the thought processes of veteran members during a response.

These scripts are offered as a method of systematically training for a wide, but typical, variety of lessons to be learned in doing CISM work. They are sprinkled throughout with almost every theme, reaction, and symptom in the book. The "Facilitator's Guide Sheet" accompanying each script contains a summary of the suggested themes, warnings about some imbedded surprises, and sample questions to guide the processing after the role play.

In some of the scenarios, there may be individuals who should not be included in the intervention. These examples can demonstrate the necessity of a good intake process to help define who should be in the debriefing/defusing. Probably most debriefers have been in a situation where one debriefee's presence has disrupted or seriously impaired the group education process. Scripting a few such common surprises is another way to improve preparedness.

SECTION 1

CISM Overview

Critical Incident Stress Management (CISM) is an integrated, comprehensive, multi-component crisis preparedness and intervention program spanning the complete crisis continuum (Everly and Mitchell, 1997). In the early days of CISM, developing teams often paid more attention to the small group components of the process. Today most CISM teams have matured into full multi-service teams. This requires those who run them, the coordinators, to become adept at "diagnosing" situations and recommending appropriate interventions from among an array of choices. Often, the advice and consultation the coordinator offers in the process of setting up services are as valuable as the interventions themselves. The task of coordinating a CISM team has become significantly more complex in recent years.

The concepts of crisis intervention and its five core competencies (pre-event strategic planning, psychological triage for affected people, one-on-one intervention, small group intervention, and large group intervention) have been evolving since 1906 when the National Save-A-Life League was formed to help prevent suicide. The experiences of military personnel during World War I and II taught us the value of providing services to adversely affected soldiers, in the vicinity of the battlefield, with the support of their friends experiencing the same event, with the understanding that they would be returned to their company quickly. The concepts of immediacy, proximity, and expectation were born here.

During the 1960s and 1970s, the evolution of crisis hotlines for suicide prevention to help people quickly through difficult times became accepted as a standard of care and an expectation for community mental health programs throughout the nation.

As research showed the value (or non-value) of each new crisis intervention strategy, it became apparent that no one strategy worked every time for every situation. Since the International Critical Incident Stress Foundation (ICISF) began in 1989, it has promoted a multi-component approach utilizing a combination of mental health and peer support personnel to provide crisis management services to first responder personnel.

Unfortunately, since an incident of workplace violence at the postal service in 1986 and the death of 13 postal workers, our country has seen a rising trend in multi-fatality incidents. Violence has not been confined to the workplace or the battlefield, but has also spread to our schools. Since September 11, 2001, our worldview has once again dramatically changed. These terrible events have challenged our society, as well as the professional community, to help the people directly and indirectly involved in these tragedies cope with the aftermath and return to daily life. Table 1.1 shows the current "state of the art" components of CISM today.

While the CISM movement has its roots in providing services to first responder personnel, it is now recognized as a standard of care for handling critical incidents in business and industry, in the military, in schools, in the religious community, and in the mental health community. It has expanded into these areas because the principles can be adapted and because it works.

Table 1.1
Critical Incident Stress Management (CISM): The Core Components

INTERVENTION	TIMING	ACTIVATION	GOAL	FORMAT
1. Pre-Crisis Preparation	Pre-crisis phase	Crisis anticipation	Set expectations. Improve coping. Stress management.	Groups and organizations
2. Demobilizations & Staff Consultation (Rescuers)	Shift disengagement	Event driven	To inform and consult, allow psychological decompression. Stress management.	Large groups and organizations
3. Crisis Management Briefing (CMB) (civilians, schools, businesses)	Anytime post-crisis			
4. Defusing	Post-crisis (within 12 hours)	Usually symptom driven	Symptom mitigation. Possible closure. Triage.	Small groups
5. Critical Incident Stress Debriefing (CISD)	Post-crisis (1-10 days; 3-4 weeks mass disasters)	Usually symptom driven, can be event driven	Facilitate psychological closure. Symptom mitigation. Triage.	Small groups
6. Individual Crisis Intervention 1:1	Anytime or anywhere	Symptom driven	Symptom mitigation. Return to function, if possible. Referral, if needed.	Individuals
7. Family CISM	Anytime	Either symptom driven or event driven	Foster support and communications.	Families and organizations
8. Community and Organizational Consultation			Symptom mitigation. Closure, if possible. Referral, if needed.	
9. Pastoral Crisis Intervention	Anytime	Usually symptom driven	To mitigate a "crisis of faith" and use spiritual tools to assist in recovery	Individuals, families or groups
10. Follow-up/Referral	Anytime	Usually symptom driven	Assess mental status. Access higher level of care, if needed.	Individuals or families

From: *Everly, G. & Mitchell, J. (1999) Critical Incident Stress Management (CISM): A New Era and Standard of Care in Crisis Intervention. Ellicott City, MD: Chevron Publishing.*

Critical Incidents vs. Crisis

What is in a name? Practically everything! One of the issues which has challenged teams is what to call themselves. This may be especially true for "in-house" teams, but it also is true for "external" teams as well. Using the term "Crisis" in a team's name denotes that it should be used only for a "CRISIS." Usually a "CRISIS" is defined by administrators as a pretty drastic event that involves death, bodily injury, or mass destruction. While that is true, there are many events that "have the power to disrupt an individual's or group's ability to cope on a temporary basis" (Mitchell & Everly, 1999) that would benefit from CISM work.

The term "Crisis Team" also denotes to many that such a team is prepared to arrive at the worksite within minutes and somehow intervene in the situation. While this may be a realistic expectation for a few types of teams (e.g., school teams), for the most part, CISM work happens *after* the event has ended. Experience has shown that the term "Crisis Team" is best avoided.

When publishing information about the team, using the phrase Critical Incident Stress Management or Critical Incident Response lends itself to a more generic opportunity to respond to events. It is important to help organizations understand that many different types of events could benefit from an appropriate CISM response other than defusing or debriefing. Table 1.2 shows some of the most common reactions that would help to identify whether or not an event is a critical incident.

Table 1.2
Common Signs and Symptoms of Excessive Stress

COGNITIVE	PHYSICAL
Confusion in thinking Difficulty making decisions Disorientation	Excessive sweating Dizzy spells Increased heart rate Rapid breathing
EMOTIONAL	**BEHAVIORAL**
Emotional shock Anger Grief Depression Feeling overwhelmed Pervading sense of hopelessness/helplessness	Changes in behavior Changes in eating Decreased personal hygiene Withdrawal from others Prolonged silences

(Adapted from Everly & Mitchell, 1995: used with permission)

The major point here is to help the leadership of the affected organization understand that many types of events are critical incidents, while only a few might be a "CRISIS."

Appropriate Responses

Does this mean that every critical incident requires that a team be called out to descend on the organization? Of course not. The whole purpose of CISM is to provide the appropriate level of response to the event. Coordinators are often asked questions such as: "Is this a critical incident? Is this something your team can help with?" The answer is not always obvious, depending as it does upon subtle factors having to do with personnel's interpretation of the meaning of the event. It is determining the reactions of the personnel of the organization that really defines a critical incident.

Experienced coordinators know that they must ask several questions of their own before they can answer. Knowing what questions to ask begins to define the art of consultation with agencies which is part of the coordinator's job. This is more fully described in Section 2, "Dispatching a Team."

Table 1.3 shows some of the most common types of events that should be considered for a CISM response. It is not an exhaustive list. The question about what you are observing from your personnel really tells the tale.

Table 1.3 Potentially Traumatizing Events

Automobile Accident Involving Injury	Major Community Disaster
Automobile Injury Involving Death	Prison Riot
Multiple Injury Accidents	Identification of Sexual Abuse
Sexual Assault	Robbery
Life Threatening Event	Suicide of Staff
Serious Physical Injury	Suicide of Child
Homicide	Suicide of Family Member
Staff Assault	Unexpected Death of Colleague
Line of Duty Death	Workplace Violence Situation
Line of Duty Injury	School Shooting
Injury of Child	Act of Terrorism
Identification of Terminal Illness	Death of a Child
Downsizing of Workplace	Hostage Situation

The Use of Peers

The makeup of CISM teams usually involves a combination of mental health trained personnel and peers from the type of organization to which the team will be providing services. Thus, CISM teams who will be working with first responders should include firefighters, law enforcement officers, nurses, and emergency services personnel. A school-based CISM team might include teachers, administrative staff, clerical staff, transportation personnel, and counselors. A team expecting to go into industrial settings would include personnel that worked in these settings.

The importance of using "peer" personnel cannot be overstated. They know the "language" of the organization being helped. They know what is a "normal" or "abnormal" situation in that industry, while a mental health person might not. Once trained, peers can be a valuable asset to both the team and the people receiving the service. Peers have "walked the walk and talked the talk." They have "been there, done that, and own the movie rights." They speak from personal experience as well as their training. They give the mental health professionals instant credibility because they are with them.

A potential pitfall for peers can be that they may revisit traumas they have been exposed to in their own work. Lacking in-depth experience in working with people after traumatic stress, they may try to "fix" their colleagues by giving advice or telling war stories of their own. They might find themselves in compromising situations and be unsure of how to avoid them or what to do when they happen. This sometimes happens when they are conducting a one-on-one and a person begins to disclose personal information that goes beyond an appropriate CISM response.

Of course, it is the commonality of their experience which makes them such a powerful authority as an intervener in the first place. One of the compelling reasons for teams to practice at every opportunity is to help all members, not just peers, form a solid sense of appropriate boundaries and practice adhering to them in a variety of situations. Providing opportunities for practice in a safe environment is a purpose of this guidebook.

Primary Purpose of CISM Activities

The primary purpose of all CISM activities is education. While CISM is indisputably an effective series of crisis intervention techniques, at its heart is the provision of information—information which other people, who have experienced a similar event, have found helpful. We believe that you must "over train" your team members with this one most important concept. Since most teams go into organizations with a fairly minimal amount of information on the group dynamics of the organization, they sometimes find themselves in very awkward situations where the debriefees have issues that go beyond the scope of a CISM team. If a team remains true to the concept that its basic mission is to provide critical incident stress management information, it can be successful in every intervention.

If team members go into a situation with the mistaken impression that they are going to "cure" everyone, or that they are going to "fix" the victims' pain, they will not last long in the CISM field because they will fail every time. If, however, they go into each situation knowing that their basic mission is to provide education and handouts, and stick to it, their intervention will be successful, even if it appears to be rejected by the participants. An example of this:

> *A team was sent to an apartment building where one of the residents had been robbed and murdered a few days earlier. The team was prepared to do a debriefing. They began with the introduction and moved to the fact phase. At this point they noticed that while there was an underlying level of anger within the group, the residents did not seem to have had a personal connection with the victim. In fact, few of the residents knew the victim and no one liked him. The major issue confronting the group was actually the loss of sense of personal safety, i.e, when was the landlord going to fix the security lights and locks on the front door, etc. The perpetrator had not been caught yet. This group still considered themselves in danger, and for them the incident was not yet over. It was definitely not time to process the aftermath of the incident.*
>
> *Instead of trying to pursue the steps of the debriefing, the team fast forwarded to the teaching phase, discussed symptoms of loss of personal safety, some things that they could do for each other and themselves, gave some quick ideas on organizing their discussion of security needs to the landlord, left handouts and information, answered questions, and left the building.*

Was this a CISM failure because the debriefing did not go well? Absolutely not. The team did not try to "force" a debriefing on a group of people who did not need it. They completed their mission by providing education on the major issues facing the group and went home. Mission accomplished successfully. The team met the needs of the group in front of them.

There may be times that a group is particularly silent or only goes to a superficial discussion of the event and self-disclosure is not forthcoming. Does the team push to make the participants "spill their guts"? Of course not. It probably means one or more of the following:

- This was not really a critical incident
- There is someone in the group that the group does not trust (in spite of careful screening prior to the defusing/debriefing)
- The event is too "raw" (are you there too early?)
- The group has had a bad experience in this type of situation in the past
- The group does not trust that the command staff didn't set up this session to "get them"
- Other unknown factors

The job of the CISM team is not to "cure" the situation. An experienced team will move relatively quickly into the teaching phase, spending more time identifying common reactions (since the group has not presented any), providing the handouts, perhaps spending a little more time "hanging out" if someone might want to approach them, and then making a follow-up phone call to see how the personnel are doing in a few days.

CISM Core Components and This Guidebook

The focus of attention of this guidebook will be on just four elements of CISM: **One-On-One Intervention, Defusings, Debriefings,** and **Crisis Management Briefings**. These interventions form the nucleus of most CISM activities. Practicing them helps CISM members build mastery and confidence in the whole range of CISM interventions. Of course, by doing this type of training and practicing, one is, in fact, also practicing pre-crisis preparation in a most practical way. Teams must receive ongoing training in all techniques to be truly useful in critical incident situations.

The first core component of CISM is **pre-crisis preparation**. A CISM team does this in a variety of ways. First, they must establish the team, decide on its mission and to whom it is willing to provide services, recruit and train volunteers, and then "market" their availability within the community they wish to serve. More detail in how to do this is covered in Section 2.

Another area that CISM teams need to address is working with the other community disaster agencies in their region. Usually a community will have a designated **Disaster Coordinator** and a written community disaster plan. This plan is often very detailed regarding how to call out and deploy personnel in the event of a natural or technological disaster, how to evacuate the community, how to direct traffic, and the entire host of details necessary to handle the immediate crisis. In many of the most elaborate, detailed plans, there is either no mention of "psychological first aid" efforts or only a few lines related to notifying Community Mental Health, the Salvation Army, the Church of the Latter Day Saints, or the local Red Cross. The assumption is that these agencies know how to do "that stuff." Sadly, this may not always be true.

At the time of any disaster or critical incident, many people in the "helping professions" will flock to the scene out of a need to help the victims. These might include religious leaders, mental health counselors, social workers, and psychologists who have excellent skills in helping others, but who are not trained in handling traumatic stress or prepared for the overwhelming pain that victims might be suffering. They can become part of the problem, rather than part of the solution, as they often attempt to do therapy rather than crisis intervention.

One of the potentially most valuable functions a CISM team might provide in a community-wide disaster is screening people who show up to provide "psychological help," but are not attached to one of the agencies designated as having a function in the disaster. This helps to protect the victims from well-meaning, but ill-trained, helpers.

The worst time to introduce a CISM team's services to the disaster coordinator is during the disaster. They do not have the time, energy, or inclination to listen to anything you might have to say, assuming that you could even speak to them. A CISM team should work with the disaster coordinator to become part of the community's disaster plan, to identify ahead of time their role and expectations, their callout planning and staging areas, and their relationship to the incident command structure.

If you are a community-based team, the community leaders must know about you *before* a critical incident. If you are prepared to work in schools, the leadership of the schools must know about you, and you must know about the rules and obligations of helping them. It will often take time to build the relationships necessary to assist in a major event. Be patient and be persistent.

The major theme here is to have connections and procedures in place *before* an event occurs. This requires pre-crisis preparation for both the team and its target population. Teams should have internal protocols written with guideline checklists, if possible. Remember, in the midst of a critical incident, chaos reigns. One of our jobs is to make sure that we are organizing the chaos to make it more manageable, and that no one falls through the cracks.

Crisis Management Briefing (CMB) is one of the latest techniques to be formalized in CISM. It is designed as a very large group intervention, usually with primary and secondary victims of an event, and it often occurs fairly quickly after the event. It differs from the other CISM group interventions both in size and scope of expectations. It does not allow the participants to talk about their experiences. Rather, it is an effort to provide education about the facts of the event, to describe the most common types of symptoms of traumatic stress that people are likely to encounter, to provide practical stress management techniques that might be helpful over the next few days, and lastly, to direct them to resources for further assistance, if necessary.

CMBs can also be used for large groups of family members of survivors of an event with a focus on teaching how they can help their loved ones. It can be used for colleagues of victims in the workplace, again with the focus on understanding what their friends might be going through and helpful techniques that they might use to assist their friends.

Having handouts that are practical and easy to understand is a requirement of all CISM responses.

A **CISM Defusing** is a brief, three-step, small-group intervention designed to provide immediate education on critical incident stress, to triage personnel after an event, and to mitigate the effects of the event. It has a paradoxical mission of both preventing the need for a debriefing, as well as making the debriefing even more powerful if held.

Teams do not practice defusings frequently enough, often assuming that if they have debriefing skills, they know how to do a defusing. While the two skills certainly build upon one another, team members need practice in both on a regular basis.

A **Critical Incident Stress Debriefing (CISD)** is a more formal, seven-step process of small group intervention for the individuals having the most direct involvement in the event, or the closest peers of the victims. The basic functions of a debriefing are to lessen the impact of the event on individuals through education, to re-establish group cohesiveness, to give permission to talk about the event with each other, and to assess the individuals or group for referral for additional assistance. It also models the opportunity to provide help and support to each other.

Individual Crisis Intervention (One-On-One) can be done in a formal or informal way. An individual can request assistance (formal) or a trained CISM team member can just "stop by to see how you are doing" (informal). The ICISF training module, "Critical Incident Stress Management (CISM): Individual Crisis Intervention and Peer Support," provides a two-day training experience and skill development on this topic.

In addition to using the basic empathy model for assisting individuals after an event, a helpful technique is to use the debriefing model questions as a method for structuring the conversation. This helps the "listener" to maintain control of the parameters of the session, keeping it focused on reactions to the event, and helps to prevent it from becoming a counseling session. The suggested statements/questions are:

- Can you tell me a little bit about what happened out there? (FACT)
- Tell me about what you were doing or saw during this situation. (FACT)
- What thought has been stuck in your head since the event was over? (THOUGHT)
- What has been the most difficult part of this for you? (REACTION)
- What have you noticed different about yourself since the event? (SYMPTOM)
- The kinds of reactions you have been describing to me are some of the most common reactions that others who have been through similar events have had. They have found it helpful to .... (TEACHING)
- So how are you doing right now? What are you going to do to take care of yourself over the next few days? (RE-ENTRY)

Using empathic listening skills during each phase lets the person talk about their experience and feel validated. Using the CISD model helps to keep the conversation on CISM and not how terrible life is, their childhood, their abusive relationships, etc. It helps to contain the conversation to CISM issues.

While **Organizational Consultation** is not a focus of this guidebook, the role-play scenarios can be used with senior leadership as a training exercise to tease out issues that the organization might address.

No use of the role plays or tabletop exercises would be complete without asking the final questions: "Is there anyone in this event that you are particularly worried about? Who might need follow-up? Who might need a referral for additional services?" This then is the component of **Follow-up/ Referral**.

SECTION 2

Operational Guidelines

This section will examine issues regarding the daily operation of CISM teams. For teams that are just getting started or for teams that have been in existence for some time, it is usually a good idea to review methods of operation on a regular basis. It is through this type of critical self-examination that coordinators assure themselves that their teams are operating effectively and efficiently.

Administrative Structure

There are many things that must be considered as a team begins to develop its operational guidelines. The first task is to determine the mission and target population of the team. Most teams have similar mission statements, but may have different target populations.

The structure of CISM teams varies widely throughout the world. Some teams become incorporated and highly organized; others follow a more leisurely and relaxed organizational development. Some have elected boards of directors, others have agency-appointed leadership responsible for the activities of the team. As with any type of organization, there are benefits to all the approaches used and some disadvantages as well. There is no "right" or "wrong" way to organize a team, provided it works well to promote the activities of the team, supports CISM principles in its work, provides for marketing of its services, and trains and supports its members.

Types of Teams

There are basically two types of teams, the "specialty" team and the "generic" team.

A **"specialty" team** is devoted to a single population of people for whom they are willing to provide CISM services. This can be the traditional first responder team, a school-based team, an "in-house" team, or any other team that focuses its efforts on a certain defined population.

A **"generic" team** is willing to provide CISM services across a broad spectrum of community events and usually has some sub-specialties within it. For example, a generic team might provide services to anyone in their community, but have first responder personnel who primarily respond to fire, police, or EMS staff, or school personnel who mainly respond to school situations. A generic team must be careful to assure that the team members responding to an event are knowledgeable about the population they will be serving. These teams are often more prevalent in smaller rural communities and offer the advantage that one community-wide training can bring CISM services into a variety of professional settings and allow for much mutual aid in the event of a community-wide incident.

Sponsorship of Teams

Once the team has determined who it is going to serve, one of the next issues to be resolved is the leadership structure and sponsorship of the team. There are three common types of sponsorship: lead-agency, agency-owned, and independent.

Many CISM teams are sponsored by a **"lead agency,"** as described by Mitchell and Everly (2001). The lead agency does not "own" the team, but often provides financial and logistical assistance. It might provide a place to meet, postage for mailings, an answering service or pager phone number, and a mailing address for the team. Lead agencies often contribute the most man-hours by providing employee time to serve as team coordinator or clinical director. When deciding on a lead agency, care must be taken to make sure that significant community "political baggage" is avoided. If a team is seen as too closely allied with a given agency, other agencies and community groups might not take advantage of the services.

Some teams are directly **"owned"** by the sponsoring agencies. This would include employee assistance program (EAP) teams, school-based teams, in-house CISM teams, or any teams that are directed under the aegis of the sponsoring agency. This team usually has a paid staff that is responsible for the development and deployment of the team. Its team members are often staff of the organization, who work with employees of their own organization or for those with which it has contracts to do CISM.

The third type of sponsorship is the "**independent team.**" This team has the advantage of not being closely allied with any community agency, but is burdened with the necessity to support itself. While the costs associated with a CISM team are usually not substantial, the team must at least provide itself with a method by which people can access the team (usually a beeper or 24-hour answering service), and must provide handouts, team brochures, and other marketing aids.

Leadership Roles

Some of the key initial **functions of the leadership** structure are:

- Identifies the goals of the team and constituency to be served
- Establishes the initial organizational structure and operational guidelines
- Obtains legal counsel to operationally define issues (if necessary)
- Provides for the financial support of the efforts and activities of the team
- Establishes the criteria for membership on the team
- Provides for the recruitment of appropriate team members
- Provides for the basic training of the team
- Creates a clear, practical operating manual
- Provides for the ongoing training of the team members
- Provides for the evaluation of team members and team activities in the field
- Provides for basic recordkeeping for the team, including both financial and team activities
- Maintains an accurate list of team members and their background (teacher, peer, mental health, clergy, etc.)

Whatever structure is ultimately decided upon, successful teams seem to have certain key ingredients, the main one being a leadership structure that includes a **Team Coordinator** function, a **Clinical Director** function, an **On-Call Coordinator** function, and an **Event Team Leader** function.

We deliberately use the term function to describe the roles, as one person might hold several roles at any given moment. For instance, the clinical director could be the on-call coordinator during a month and decide to function as the event team leader on a particular response during the month. It is important that the functions be clearly delineated and that they are divided among various people to avoid over-burdening individual team members.

The **Team Coordinator** functions as the CEO of the organization. This person's responsibility is to run the team meetings, organize the agenda, and to serve as the "spark plug" for keeping the team operating. Team coordinators often share responsibility for most of the administrative functions, e.g., recruiting and screening members, communication within the team, conducting meetings, etc. They are often the team's most visible representative and perform much of the pre-crisis preparation, marketing, etc. They assume responsibility for continuing education and general "care and feeding" of the team. For example, it is usually the coordinator's job to make sure that a "debriefing of the debriefers" is held after every response. And finally, coordinators keep records and conduct outcome assessments.

The **Clinical Director** is one of the mental health professionals on the team. He or she works closely with the team coordinator to ensure that the team functions smoothly, assists in developing the team protocols, and usually is responsible for overseeing the training of the team.

The clinical director makes sure that team members are both adequately trained and carry out their responsibilities within their scope of professional practice. The clinical director may at times be called upon to evaluate the performance of individual team members and to provide clinical supervision for enhancement of their skills. Usually the clinical director and team coordinator work together to provide for the overall functioning of the team. They frequently represent the team in public or as part of a regional or state association. They promote the activities of the team among the populations the team is supporting and often are involved with the general "marketing "of the team.

The third major function in a CISM team that is often shared among several experienced people to prevent "burnout" is the role of the **On-Call Coordinator**. This person has the primary responsibility for:

1. Taking the call from the person requesting a response, obtaining all the necessary information to evaluate the significance of the incident, and determining what the appropriate level of response might be.
2. Educating and consulting with the person requesting the services about the reactions being described and possible courses of action that can be taken. This could include referral to other resources, giving additional information on what the team does or does not do, arranging the timing of the interventions, and determining who might be invited.
3. Notifying the organization as to the needs of the team (space requirements, refreshments, quiet area, members taken out of service, etc.).
4. Recruiting team members to accomplish the intervention.
5. Organizing the response with the requesting agency (adequate room, personnel out of service, food and beverages available, etc.).
6. Assuring that a debriefing of the debriefers is held.
7. Documenting the response.

In some team models, the on-call coordinator also goes to the debriefing site, but is not directly involved in the service. The on-call coordinator is then available to "trouble shoot" any problems and to actually lead the debriefing of the debriefers.

It is strongly recommend that the on-call coordinator position be rotated among several senior/experienced members of the team on a monthly basis, so that no one is overly burdened by the experience. After all, critical incidents happen at all times of the day and night, including on holidays.

The **Event Team Leader** is the team member who is appointed to be in charge of the response in the field. Sometimes the on-call coordinator will choose to fill this role him/herself. At other times an experienced member will be assigned the role. Necessary experience includes at least two previous responses to this type of event. For example, a member who has at least two previous defusings may be chosen to be the event team leader for a defusing. His/her duties will include consulting with administration, assessment of further needs, leading the response itself, ensuring a team debriefing sometime afterwards, and recordkeeping for the coordinator. This person is entrusted to be flexible and to adapt to the unexpected. If a response must be changed or even terminated prematurely, it would be the responsibility of the event team leader to do so.

Suggested Committees

Usually teams will also have a need for some committees to assist in the overall functioning of the team. These often include a **Recruitment Committee** to seek, interview, evaluate, and welcome new team members. It is important that teams recruit new people and ideas so they do not become stagnant. It is also of great benefit to make sure new members are quickly brought into the workings of the team and made to feel an active part of the team.

Experienced recruiters often begin with a strategy of calling for volunteers following an in-service presentation, but eventually gravitate towards a more proactive strategy of seeking out those who have the requisite "people skills" of a "natural" CISM member. This is because there are so many motives for volunteering for such work, not all of which correlate with the abilities to do it. Those involved with recruiting and screening over a period of time generally develop their own list of characteristics of a "natural," e.g., respected by peers, people skills, low-maintenance ego, can keep a secret, etc.

Depending upon the team structure, an **Education Committee** is often helpful. This committee serves two major functions: it supports and helps to provide for the on-going training of the team and often serves as a "marketing" committee by providing education to the agencies the team serves. In its team education role, it might provide for an annual in-house training seminar or a 20- to 30-minute presentation at team meetings. The committee can provide handouts on the latest CISM research or materials. It might provide a "mentoring" program for new team members as they are gaining the skills necessary to do CISM work.

In its "marketing role," the education committee might provide for team members to go to staff meetings of local units to teach an overview of critical incident stress or about the services of the team and how to contact it (pre-incident education). Many first responder organizations require that their membership gain additional training in stress management. The CISM team can often provide that training for the department and then talk about the team as well. Another example of the work of this committee is to speak to the leadership of the organizations to be served and to provide appropriate materials for handouts and methods to access the CISM team. Without this ongoing pre-incident education, organizations are less likely to think of your team as a resource in difficult times.

These two types of subcommittees appear to be present in most teams that last over time. They provide ways for the team to maintain an active role in their community, bring in new members who may have fresh ideas and replace personnel who leave, and lastly, help to assure that the team maintains adequate resources to do its work within the community to which it has dedicated itself.

Team Size

How many team members does a team need to function well? There is no easy correct answer to this question. The ideal is to have enough members to be able to respond to all requests for services without over-burdening individual team members. Since most team members are volunteers, they can say "no" to requests that come during inconvenient times and can leave the team at any time. It is not unusual to hear an on-call coordinator tell of making dozens of phone calls before recruiting a three-person response team. However, it is also undesirable to have so many members that some people do not get called out for months at a time, if ever. Experience will be the ultimate teacher, but there is a method for estimating a team's critical size.

First, through research or guesswork, estimate the frequency of critical incidents in your target population. Count only the ones to which your group would be likely to respond. Then pick a number of responses per year to which you would be comfortable inviting any particular member. This may involve how much tolerance for work-release time members have, as well as their personal tolerance for stress. How many responses per year can the average person do and still be comfortable? If you are planning a team for a small fire department which has about three or four incidents per year, and you feel members can easily do three responses per year, then you could probably get by with two mental health and three to six peer members. On the other hand, a community-based "generic" team serving a small city and having a base-rate of 24 responses per year has a critical size of about 40 members, with the expectation of only two responses per year for most members. Similarly, in-house teams in prisons or psychiatric hospitals may respond to several events per week and may require much larger teams.

Team Records

One of the keys to preventing burnout (besides debriefing the debriefers, which will be discussed later) is keeping good records on the team's activities and who has been called and who has not been called to assist with a response. Coordinators frequently prefer to work with people they know and trust, so often the same people are the first ones called. This prevents newer members from gaining experience and they may drop out because they are not being utilized. At the same time, the personnel who are always used may drop out from exhaustion. Doing CISM is hard work, and people need time to recover after participating in a response. Good recordkeeping helps to ensure equal use of all members.

Keeping good records on individual team members' responses also helps to build team leadership. You generally want some of your most experienced personnel serving in the on-call coordinator position. Keeping track of your team members' experiences helps you cultivate new leadership and makes sure that newer members are properly mentored. Most teams have adopted a method to keep track of individual membership by name, occupation/specialty, phone number, address, and date of joining the team. The more sophisticated teams also try to track how frequently the person has been utilized (or even just called), any types of events that the person should not be called for (either because of personal choice or new life circumstance), etc. A team also frequently needs to keep an "inactive reserve" list. A person may be put on inactive status because they recently had a loss in their personal life (death of a family member, divorce, or loss of job), because they had an addition to their life (birth of a child, recently married, or changed jobs), or simply because they ask to be placed on the inactive list. The golden rule, "first, do no harm," applies to teammates as well as to the public.

It is important to keep good records of the training attended by individual members. This identifies your most experienced personnel and those members who have had advanced training. This again helps in "mentoring" and modeling for newer members and also allows you to pick appropriate members to handle different types of events.

Meetings

How often should a team meet? Once a year is too seldom and once a week is probably too frequent, so the ideal time is somewhere in between. In the beginning stages, most teams seem to meet at least monthly to get organized and to get up and running. In the beginning, there is much work to be done. However, after the first year or two, most of the necessary details are in place and having meetings three or four times per year is probably sufficient. However, regular meetings are necessary. They should be short, efficient, and fun. Do not waste people's time or they will stop coming. Never hold a meeting without providing some type of training experience. Team members need some reasons to attend meetings.

Standard agenda items might include:

- Introduction of members present and welcoming of new members
- Review of any responses made since the previous meeting and lessons learned (let the members tell their experiences)
- Report on the financial health of the team
- Report on the activities of the recruitment committee
- Report on the activities of the educational committee
- Any additional agenda items
- A brief educational experience such as a video, a new handout, new material put out by ICISF, review of procedures for handling a CISM response, or one of the activities described in Section 3 of the manual

Membership Application and Screening

This is an area where a team can be very formal or quite informal. A team does not want to be seen as exclusive or elite, but at the same time it is important that the team has confidence in its members before dispatching them to do CISM work. Most successful teams incorporate the following steps in the process:

1. **Basic Requirements**
   - Applicants should receive training in the ICISF Basic CISM model
     —Some teams require an ICISF certified training
     —Some teams also require a combination of training and "on the job" experience of working several times with a CISM team in the field
2. **Screen the Applicants**
   - A screening process that requires a review and sponsorship of the individual
     —This usually includes an interview with the applicant to determine their background and interest in CISM
     —It is usually a good idea to see if anyone on the current team knows the applicant and can give feedback or provide a reference
3. **Mentoring Program**
   - A "mentoring" program that pairs a "seasoned" team member with a new member
     —The mentor makes sure the person knows the basics of how the team operates and serves as their initial "best buddy," introducing them to other team members and making sure they feel comfortable at their first team meetings
     —When possible, the mentor tries to make sure that the new person is included in a field assignment in the first month or two that they are active on the team
4. **On-The-Job Training**
   - A process by which the new team member gains experience and gets feedback from the event team leader, coordinator, or clinical director

These steps help to maintain an adequate supply of team members and build the quality of the team.

Initial Training

The ideal standard, recommended by ICISF, is three certified trainings—Basic, Individual (Peer), and Advanced CISM—a total of six days of training in all. A member with these trainings would be prepared to handle most of the CISM interventions needed in any situation. Standardized training in CISM assures greater consistency in providing services and assists team members in working with each other during interventions. Of course, we all know debriefers with years of experience in every conceivable situation and only basic CISM training. Teams have limitations, budgetary constraints, manpower shortages, and geographical isolation. In an attempt to make standardized trainings available almost anywhere, ICISF has created a cadre of certified trainers. But even in the most affluent organizations, the usual situation is that just a few key members have three or more ICISF trainings under their belt, while many others do not. One of the premises of this manual is that the most experienced and best-trained members, often coordinators, will be expected to pass on their expertise through local continuing education and internal trainings.

If possible, all team members should go through a certified two-day *Critical Incident Stress Management (CISM) or Basic Group Crisis Intervention* course as promoted by the International Critical Incident Stress Foundation. This course gives the basis for doing all CISM small group work. Any and all additional coursework regarding CISM is also encouraged.

After the initial basic training, team members should be introduced to practicing the CISM models by utilizing the "2+2+2" model of learning: observe 2, practice 2, and assist on 2 for each type of intervention. For example, they should observe two role-plays or videos of debriefings to see the model, they should practice at least two debriefing role plays, and should assist on two actual CISD experiences before being put in a position of leadership within a CISD response.

This model allows a new team member to gain substantial exposure to the models of CISM interventions before being called upon to do any facilitation themselves. New team members start by leading the FACT phase in their first few debriefings. This allows them to participate, but in a phase of the debriefing where they are not called upon to do much interpretation of what they are hearing.

Team coordinators should know the exact experience-base of all members. Dispatching teams with the appropriate experience-base for the demands of a particular situation is part of the art of coordinating a CISM team. The team dispatched to an incident involving accidental fatalities is not the same team dispatched to the aftermath of an event like the September 11th terrorist attacks. The relevant question in attempting to define training standards is not: "What is an acceptable training/experience level for CISM work?" but rather, "What is an acceptable training/experience level for this type of situation?"

Team leaders inevitably develop their own answers to that question over time. They are influenced by professional opinions about generally accepted standards of practice and by more practical factors like limitations in local resources, training budgets, etc. The following table is offered to answer the question of adequate training for different situations.

Type of Situation	Acceptable Training/Experience	Competencies
Any CISM (back-up only team member)	2-day basic training in CISM, preferably by a certifying organization or equivalent	Knows the model being used
Any CISM work where people are helped	Basic training, including 2 observations and 2 role plays	Assessment; one-on-one small group intervention
Coordinate a CISM team	Basic training and additional (advanced/specialty) training and several responses	Large group interventions; strategic planning
Major disaster	Basic training and other special training (preferably disaster), plus 5 responses or several years experience	

Appendix #1 provides sample questions that are asked in the ICISF "Model for Debriefing." These can be placed on index cards and laminated as training aids and prompts for new debriefers.

Dispatching a Team Into the Field

The phone/beeper goes off and you respond. The first words you hear are "We need a debriefing!" What is your next step? It is not to start making calls to gather together a team to go running off to do "a debriefing." The coordinator's job is to assess what services are most indicated, and through consultation with the "management," agree upon a plan. When serving a particular work location for the first time, it is often best to do this consultation on-site, especially if your recommendation is to delay services longer than requested.

Experienced coordinators work from a checklist of questions that serve as memory prompts to aid assessment. At this stage of the "state-of-the-art" in CISM, there is not much standardization of these checklists. Most coordinators develop their own favorite list. An example is offered in the Appendix 2 titled simply, "Questions Coordinators Ask." The first six groups of questions help a coordinator **analyze the situation** enough to suggest appropriate choices from the list of CISM interventions and begin to plan the timing and personnel of responses. These are questions often asked by the team coordinator, or more likely, the on-call coordinator. The last group of questions helps the on-call coordinator or even the event team leader **analyze the group** itself enough to avoid unwelcome surprises. A few of these latter questions are often asked on-site, just before a response, as a sort of last check. A sample format for actually capturing the information from the questions can be found in Appendix 4.

There are some surprises you do not want to walk into when conducting a response. And after you do it once, a question gets added to your list so that you do not walk into that surprise ever again. Surprises such as a hot union grievance, sub-grouping, anger or blaming within the group, a known procedural mistake causing the incident, or a manager who mistakenly thinks he or she is "one of the guys" can put a team in some awkward situations which would be better avoided or at least prepared for. Another on-call coordinator's job, then, is to avoid surprises. Some such surprises can leave participants feeling worse than before they came—not a good outcome. Remember, it is not the team's job to fix the organization's pre-existing problems.

As a group process, any CISM intervention has three goals:

- To provide a safe environment for the participants to talk about the event and their reactions to it **(provide for ventilation)**
- To provide the opportunity for individuals to have their thoughts and feelings validated by other members of the group **(provide for validation)**
- To provide encouragement for individuals to support each other **(provide for validation)**
- To teach CISM techniques **(provide for education)**

It is just as important to be able to define what an intervention *is not*, as it is to define what it is. In the area of consultation with agencies, having a clear sense of boundaries for your team's mission is crucial. Many administrators will not know enough about CISM to have a realistic idea of what your activities can and cannot accomplish. It is one of the challenges of good coordinating to be able to define your boundaries clearly. Whether involved in consultation, or in leading an intervention, effective CISM members remember the boundary suggested by the negative three **F**'s of good listening: "Don't **F**eed it, Don't **F**ight it, and Don't **F**ix it."

Don't feed it means that debriefers do not encourage individuals to overexpose personal data or engage in negative comments about the situation or organization. Individuals who have been exposed to a critical incident may seek someone or some organization to blame for the event.

This is counterproductive as it allows them to avoid addressing their personal reaction to the event. The debriefers should restate from the introduction that it is not the purpose of the intervention to blame or find fault.

Don't fight it suggests that the debriefers should avoid arguing or trying to use logic to change the opinions of the debriefees.

Don't fix it recognizes that the debriefers are working as facilitators to assist the participants in talking about the event and hearing that their reactions are normal reactions of normal people who have experienced an abnormal event. Any meaningful "fixing" will come from within the individuals and/or the group. It is not our task to "fix" pre-existing organizational problems.

> *A CISM team of three is dispatched to debrief third shift staff at a psychiatric hospital after one of the staff had committed suicide. The coordinator, seeing this assessment of need as a no-brainer, asks all the dispatching type questions (16 people, etc.), but neglects to ask what kind of a group this is. The team leader recounted later that he began to suspect a problem when five debriefees remained standing along the wall and consistently refused to join the circle. It turns out that the staff had been split down the middle for some time because of a year-long labor dispute, to the point of some personal animosities and car vandalization. One of the sub-groups was so angry that they actively blamed management for their friend's suicide. The team leader reflected that the few minutes it took them to figure out what was going on and agree to end the group "seemed like a lot longer." Afterwards, the manager who had made the request told the CISM coordinator "I thought it might do them good, maybe get over some differences, and besides, you didn't ask." Another question goes on the coordinator's list.*

Ask ten coordinators to list the **main functions** of their job and you might get ten different lists. But they would all include these elements:

- Assess the need for *any* of the ten CISM components
- Assess the group dynamics and the situation to avoid surprises
- Put the right CISM providers together for this population and situation
- Re-assess periodically through follow-up and outcome
- Provide for the "care and feeding" of the team (supervision, etc.)

At any point in the life of a CISM response, the coordinator's re-assessment might prompt the addition of any of the ten components to CISM work (see Table 1.1):

Pre-Incident Preparation
- Demobilizations
- Crisis Management Briefings
- Defusing
- Debriefing
- Individual Crisis Intervention (One-on-One)
- Family CISM
- Community and Organizational Consultation
- Pastoral CISM
- Follow-up and Referral

The first basic task of the on-call coordinator is to gather enough information so the most appropriate intervention can be selected and implemented. Some of the initial questions to be asked are:

- What was the event?
- How many personnel were involved? From what departments?
- What are observations of the effect on personnel?
- How many seem to be affected?
- Does the leadership of the affected organization know about and support this request?

These first five questions begin to determine what type of response the CISM team might make to the situation. Although the first question about the type and duration of the event is an important one, it does not automatically determine whether the event is a critical incident. It is, in fact, the third question that begins to tell the tale: "What are you seeing from your personnel?" Remember, a critical incident is any event that has the power to disrupt an individual or group's ability to cope on a temporary basis.

Some events by their very nature are almost always a critical incident. Things like a line of duty death or severe injury, death or severe injury to children, or a particularly difficult or horrific scene are often automatic triggers for a defusing or debriefing response. But, since personnel sometimes interpret events differently, it is really the description of their reactions to the event that demonstrates the need for a response, as well as the type and size of response.

It is also important to mention here that what is viewed by one group as a critical incident may not be viewed by another group as anything out of the ordinary. EMS personnel often dismiss sights at an accident scene involving a casualty which would keep most of the rest of us up for several nights. But what is a coordinator to do about two first-responder agencies involved in the same incident but disagreeing about the need for CISM services? The answer is that this happens on an individual basis all the time. We handle it by referring to the introductory comment which asks those who don't feel they need this service to stay as a support to their coworkers. The coordinator starts a dialogue between the command personnel of the two agencies, exploring whether a joint response is possible, otherwise known as consultation.

It is also critically important to know who is making the request and whether or not the person calling is authorized by the leadership to do so. The team which shows up without an authorized invitation could be in for one of those awkward surprises which have the potential to make a situation worse. Another question goes on the coordinator's list (Appendix 2).

If a response is appropriate, the next set of questions begins to structure it. You might ask questions like:

- How urgent is the situation?
- How many people are expected to be there?
- The mandatory vs. voluntary question
- Where can the session(s) be held? (explain about sitting in a circle, someplace quiet, etc.)
- How to get there? (get good directions; your team doesn't need the stress of being lost)
- Can all personnel be taken out of duty during the response?
- When can you get back with the person to confirm?

Coordinators are often asked whether employees' attendance at a response should be mandatory or voluntary. There are several organizational factors which may dictate this decision, e.g., contract restrictions on working hours, the agency's ability to keep employees "on-the-clock," etc. But all of those aside, the best advice seems to be that a manager should make attendance mandatory, or at least "highly encouraged," and trust the team to make participation voluntary. If there is good reason to believe people will be adversely impacted, then there is good reason to treat everyone's risk preventatively. Besides, most CISM veterans have observed that often those who were most exposed to risk factors are the ones who avoid services the most. Sometimes, if this seems likely, the manager is advised to seek out these employees for a personal invitation or extra bit of "encouragement."

At this point, the on-call coordinator has determined what type of response is required and begins to orchestrate the response. The on-call coordinator must explain to the requesting agency what the team needs when they arrive:

- A place to meet with the leadership/host before the response begins
- A place to meet with the personnel
- Some appropriate refreshments for the re-entry phases (fruit juices, healthy foods, etc.)

While the emphasis on promoting healthy refreshments immediately after an incident is good, for some agencies coffee is a continual need, and the team is a guest in their agency, so do not push it too hard.

The requesting agency's management should be advised to consider inviting personnel from any other departments that were on scene who might have been affected by the incident. At this time, arrangements should be made for a return phone call or visit before the response begins.

Most requests and determinations are made over the phone, but occasionally, especially if responding to a community organization, it is beneficial to meet at the organization to plan the response. This gives the on-call coordinator the opportunity to see firsthand what the needs are, what the agency might be like, and to establish the guidelines for the team's response. Oftentimes, community organizations may not clearly understand what CISM services are and may need more explanation prior to bringing staff in for CISM services.

The on-call coordinator then begins to assemble a team to respond. Each team should include one mental health professional and peers of the agency or agencies requesting the service. This is where good recordkeeping is again very important. It is helpful if the on-call coordinator knows who is experienced, who has a background in the type of event or agency that has been affected by the incident, who needs additional "seasoning," and who might head up this team.

Once the team is identified, it is a good idea to establish one of the more senior persons as the event team leader. In this role, one of the team members is in charge for this particular response and takes the lead in seeing that the team performs its responsibilities during the response, and that it gets a debriefing of the debriefers at the end of the work. Sometimes, an event team leader is not the most experienced person, but someone who is being "seasoned" for future leadership on the team. The more experienced personnel can provide feedback to the leader at the end of the response.

It is usually up to the event team leader to connect with the requesting agency to confirm the plans and to obtain any additional information needed before arrival at the site. These final questions concentrate on any last-minute developments and on getting a clearer picture of the group with which the team will be working. Any details about the participants, their mix, or their issues will help the team be sensitive to the culture of the organization they are visiting. As mentioned above, avoiding surprises is a worthy goal for an event team leader (Appendix 2).

It is the responsibility of the event team leader to "brief" the team as to all the issues known prior to arriving at the site. This includes the type of event, the primary issues expected to be heard by the team, and in short, any and all information they need to do a good job. This is usually a good time to decide upon any team roles for the event or who is going be doing what in the CISM intervention selected for this event.

It is usually a good idea to arrive at the service site at least 30 minutes before the activities are scheduled to begin. The team meets with the leadership/host and again goes over what the event was, who is scheduled to come to the site, and asks some final questions about recent developments and the make-up of the group.

- Is there any new information about the event?
- Who was closest to the victim?
- What have personnel being doing in the interim?
- What are they talking most about?
- Is there any blaming going on?
- Do you have any questions about what we are going to be doing here today?

This is the last time the team gets to hear any information that might affect its work prior to actually beginning it. Depending upon the answers to such questions, the team might decide that they are going to be doing different work than had been originally prepared.

The team might provide a combination of debriefing and individual work if that is the most appropriate service. They may have come prepared to do a crisis management briefing only to find the needs are for a regular critical incident stress debriefing. While good preparation helps to reduce the number of surprises, the team must maintain a flexible approach to providing CISM services.

Readers are directed to Appendices 2 and 4 for a format that helps to capture some of the information discussed above. It has proven to be a good starting point for teams to develop their own checklists of assessment and consultation questions.

Debriefing the Debriefers

A special type of supervision is the peer-supervision provided in a team format by the process defined as **Debriefing the Debriefers**. The standard of practice these days dictates that, especially after difficult events, CISM teams be assembled again some time after a response to go through a debriefing of their own. It is during this experience that any concerns about their individual performances are discussed and prevented from becoming a residual problem by the peer support inherent to the model.

Although simply a truncated version of the seven-stage ICISF model, a team debriefing has one important difference. Unlike a regular debriefing, a team debriefing *does* have a critique component. Team members do not just experience a response; they facilitate it. In doing their work, members put their professional egos on the line. Their judgments about how they performed professionally are crucial to their experience of stress and should be explored in the supportive confines of group supervision for the event team.

The Model

Some teams evolve strategies for trying to make sure no one becomes overwhelmed with doing too much too often. These are important parts of a CISM team protocols, but they are not enough. From the earliest beginnings of the ICISF work, taking care of team members has been recognized as important, but no standard model for caring for the team had evolved.

The debriefing the debriefers model was developed to put some structure to the process and has become a standard operating procedure after each event. The model is offered as a basis for helping your team members recover from their work.

Why Do It?

When a CISM team has finished its work with the personnel involved in a critical incident, they are normally tired and ready to return to their own lives. They can often be described as being in a state of "excited exhaustion" where their minds are racing and excited by the work of the intervention, but their energy level is depleted. However, they still have one piece of work left to be done, namely, to take a few minutes to take care of themselves.

Because the team has spent several hours being exposed to the pain of the personnel involved in the event, they too have become participants in it. As a result, team members may have some reactions to the debriefing, a process called vicarious traumatization.

The process of debriefing the debriefers attempts to accomplish three goals:

- To **prevent** negative reactions such as vicarious traumatization, cumulative stress, and the effects of negative self-judgment
- To **teach and reinforce skills** demonstrated during the debriefing
- To "**practice what we preach**" with members of the team

By assuring that a debriefing of the debriefers is a standard operating procedure for your team, you are increasing members' effectiveness and longevity on the team. You are decreasing the chances for any negative personal reactions by members of the team and monitoring the team for any adverse reactions. Lastly, like the debriefees, the team is being prepared for re-entry into their "normal" world.

Typically, the debriefing should be done shortly after their work is finished and if possible, before the team separates to go home. If a team has been involved in a particularly difficult debriefing or a series of defusings/debriefings/demobilizations during a prolonged event response, the debriefing might be more appropriate within a few days or a week later. This will allow the team an opportunity to process some of the event on their own and then to finish the work together.

The debriefing the debriefers process normally takes 15 to 30 minutes for "regular" debriefings and longer for particularly difficult or long interventions.

Who Should Do It?

Usually the event team leader or an experienced peer can lead the debriefing debriefers process. If the debriefing team has been through a particularly difficult or long response, their debriefing is best accomplished by someone who was not a direct part of the response. This allows all team members to participate in the full experience of the debriefing process. It also allows for "fresh eyes and ears" to provide feedback and teaching to the team. Team coordinators often fill this role.

How Do You Do It?

The debriefing debriefers process uses a variation of the ICISF model. It consists of three phases **review**, **response**, and **remind**.

The **review** phase is essentially a combination of the introduction/fact/thought phase of the regular debriefing. It utilizes questions designed to have members think about and discuss the debriefing and their participation in it. The following questions are prompts for this phase:

- How did it go?
- How do you think you did?
- What themes emerged?
- What was the participation level of the group?
- Is there anything you are worried about?

During this phase, the leader can guide the discussion into teaching what made the response go well or give examples of other ways to have handled some aspect of it.

The **response** phase is a condensation of the reaction/symptom phase of the ICISF model and works to elicit comments on the self-perception of the team members and any concerns they may have about their performance. The following types of questions seem to work well:

- What did you say that you wish you hadn't?
- What didn't you say that you wish you had?
- How has this debriefing affected you?
- What was the most difficult part of this debriefing for you?
- Is there anything you did that you're concerned about?

During this phase, the leader guides some group discussion of the members' self-impressions. If team members are blaming themselves for something, or worried that they did something really wrong, it usually comes out during this phase. What then usually follows is reassurance by the fellow team members that no major errors occurred. This is also an opportunity for the team leader and team members to reassure each other that each individual contributed to the process and to offer alternative methods for handling problem issues. This is a prime time to teach new techniques or reinforce lessons learned.

The **remind** phase correlates to the teaching/re-entry phase of the Mitchell model. Questions in this step serve to help the team remember to do the same sort of things that we encourage the debriefees to do.

- Is there any follow up to be done?
- What are you going to do to take care of yourself in the next 24 hours?
- What will it take for you to "let go" of this debriefing?

Where To Do It?

Any neutral site that provides enough privacy is appropriate for this process. Team members should be able to relax and discuss thoughts confidentially and without interruptions. The more difficult the CISM responses were, the more privacy is needed.

If the team has been on a particularly difficult debriefing or event, one last piece of education can be given to them. It can be suggested that they "make up two stories" about the event they have just worked. One is the "Readers' Digest" version to be given in general to people who might ask, and the other is the more complete version identifying how their participation might have affected them. While neither version should violate any confidentiality of the event, having the two stories allows the debriefer to safely answer questions from close friends and loved ones quickly.

By using this structured approach to debriefing debriefers, CISM teams are maximizing the opportunities for teaching members new skills, minimizing the chances for members returning home distressed or full of self-doubt, and assuring its members that they are valuable assets to the team. Being involved in a CISM team ought to be a rewarding experience for all team members. It is our responsibility to take care of ourselves at least as well as we try to take care of others.

Table 2.1
DEBRIEFING THE CISM TEAM

Analogous Phases of CISD	**Three-Phase Debriefing of CISM Teams (Sample Questions)**	**Goals**
FACT	I. REVIEW —How did it go? —Were the participants active? —What themes emerged? —How do you think you did? —Any surprises?	COMPARE FACTS/ THOUGHTS VENTILATION
REACTION/ SYMPTOM	II. RESPONSE —How have you been feeling about this one? —What was the most difficult aspect of this debriefing? —Anything you wish you had handled better?	VALIDATION/ MUTUAL SUPPORT/ SUPERVISION
TEACHING/ RE-ENTRY	III. REMIND —Any follow-up to be done? —What is one thing you learned from this? —Is there anything you need to "let go" of? —What are you going to do to take care of yourself in the next 24 hours?	EDUCATION/ CONSOLIDATION/ STRESS MANAGEMENT

Other Techniques

The model described in Table 2.1 is offered as one good technique for team maintenance. But, of course, there are others, which include:

- Follow-up phone calls to provide private processing time
- Telling stories and relating experiences at regular meetings
- Journaling or reporting about lessons learned
- Skill building games and exercises
- Role playing, especially concerning special challenges

Handouts

During every CISM response, handouts should be distributed. There are many sources for handouts, and probably every team uses a variation of one developed by Jeffrey T. Mitchell as its basic, all-purpose handout. But just as CISM has matured and expanded in its range of responses, so too must a team expand its available handouts.

A team should begin to collect or develop handouts for the types of responses and the groups of people for whom they are responding. Handouts of one or two pages that cover topics of general grief, suicide, talking with loved ones after a critical incident, talking with children about death, what to say after a disaster, or how to talk to the family members of the deceased are all topics used frequently during CISM work.

Specialty teams such as school-based teams should have a wide assortment of handouts available for school staff and parents.

The International Critical Incident Stress Foundation has sample handouts available on their Web site (www.icisf.org) that cover many topics for first responder personnel. Kantu Consultants also maintains some handout material on our Web page (www.Kantu.org). Other related Internet sites frequently have good handout materials as well.

Teams should not overwhelm participants with too many handouts. However, leaving some behind based upon the issues raised during the course of the CISM services is a great teaching device. Personnel can read them at leisure, perhaps when they are most needed and you are not around.

Referrals for Additional Service

On rare occasions, someone may request additional assistance that goes beyond the educational function of CISM services. This can be a tricky issue to handle for the team. If a referral is going to be made (and if one should be requested), the following are key issues to be considered:

- What is the need of the person requesting additional help?
- Is it for something especially troubling from the critical incident?
- Is it for something more generic like marriage counseling or individual therapy because of other life situations?
- Is the person having a significant crisis that requires immediate professional help? (Are they thinking of suicide? Homicide?)

If the need is for help in dealing with life's general issues of loss and problems, it is probably safe to give the person a list of mental health agencies in the community that provide these types of services. However, if it is specifically related to a critical incident, the general mental health practitioner may have little training in crisis response or posttraumatic stress disorder (PTSD). If a first responder is asking for additional help, few general mental health practitioners will have experience or understanding in the special on-the-job stressors associated with this line of work.

Some of the experienced mental health personnel in this field may be members of the CISM team. Making referrals to these people makes a great deal of sense, but at the same time raises issues of the mental health personnel "padding their practice" by such referrals. The team must make sure they are doing nothing to give the appearance of impropriety.

Since every community is different in the resources it may have available for providing therapy to persons who have experienced a critical incident, teams should research local providers and have lists of choices available. The team must take care in making referrals to make sure no member is taking advantage of his/her position on the team. It is also a good idea to ask about employee benefits so that if the subject comes up, the team can remind employees how to access help. All of these above decisions might be said to involve "triage," and are often the role of the mental health team member.

Monitoring Team Members' Performance

We all come to CISM services from a variety of backgrounds and for a variety of reasons. Hopefully, everyone who joins a CISM team has, as their basic motivation, a desire to help people who have experienced a critical incident. Almost always this is true...*almost* always.

Some start out with this desire, but somewhere along the road they may change. Sometimes people begin to confuse service to others with service to their own egos. Some really like the adrenaline rush that comes with crisis work. Some people, in spite of their commitment and good motivations, may simply lack the ability to do the work. A team needs to know its members and the quality of the work they do. A team needs the ability to monitor and correct the behavior of its members. While some of the screening procedures described earlier in this section may help to prevent people from joining the team for inappropriate reasons, they will not catch all of them, nor do they catch the "changeling." There are several elements involved in monitoring team members' performance:

- Team "memo of understanding" (that specifies expectations)
- Team rules (written and given to each team member)
- Observation and supervision during practice exercises
- Supervision during responses (mentoring, peer-supervision, debriefing of team)
- Clear process for "request for evaluation" of a team member

The memo of understanding serves to establish the expectations for team members and illustrates appropriate team behavior in general terms. Appendix 3 provides a sample format.

While not every single team needs an extensive operations manual, it is a good idea to have some written documentation that outlines the mission of the team, perhaps some guiding principles, and in general describes appropriate team behavior. This might include the do's and don'ts for members.

Lastly, there should be a clear process that allows any team member to request an evaluation of another member's performance. This might come about because a team member made significant mistakes during a response, has violated team rules, or in some fashion has done something that has the potential for damaging a team's reputation. Some examples might be:

- A breech of confidentiality
- Failure to follow CISM or team protocols
- Providing team CISM services without team permission
- Using the membership on the team to advance one's personal agenda
- Misrepresenting their position within the team
- Being convicted of a crime

Each team must develop its own set of disciplinary standards. These often include a vote of the selected leadership or the establishment of a committee to evaluate the situation and make recommendations to the leadership for action.

In the situation where a member seems to lack the skills necessary to carry out their responsibilities, it is usually the clinical director's responsibility to sit in on and observe the work of the member, to provide for additional training opportunities, and eventually to recommend the continuation or termination of membership on the team.

There are also many important roles on a CISM team that do not entail providing direct services. These can be roles that are filled with personnel who do not participate in debriefings, defusings, or other direct-service activities of the team but do support the team and its members through other roles, perhaps on the education or recruitment committees. Members who temporarily put themselves on the temporary inactive list (perhaps because of a personal life crisis) often are willing to turn their energies to some of these activities.

Monitoring the performance of a volunteer team member is not always enjoyable work. However, to maintain the integrity, reputation, and viability of the team, every team needs to know that it can trust its members to do good work.

Recordkeeping

Recordkeeping for a CISM team is usually pretty minimal, but keeping the right *kind* of records can help insure the longevity of a team in several ways:

- Prevent either burnout or stagnation by ensuring equal use of members
- Prevent disinterest by keeping members informed of team activities
- Provide feedback and reinforcement to sponsoring agencies
- Provide a quality control function by identifying members who need extra supervision or have various skills

A team's records should focus on the team itself and its issues, not the population served. This is primarily to protect the confidentiality of the service population. Ideally, a team's records should be able to answer the following questions:

- How many incidents have been responded to?
- What groups have been served?
- How many people have received your services?
- Of all the CISM services, how many of which types were provided (i.e., how many defusings, debriefings, individual contacts, etc.)?
- Where is each team member in his or her training/experience sequence (i.e., how many observations, role plays, defusing, debriefings, etc.)?
- What are each team member's current strengths, weaknesses, or special skills (e.g., do you note who just had a death in their family; who is bilingual; who is best with certain groups; who should be on an "inactive" list, etc.)?
- Who should get the first call for the next response?

A note about the inactive list: not all teams keep such a list formally, but there are good reasons for a team coordinator or clinical director to keep brief notes regarding the changing life circumstances of team members. CISM work can be demanding, and we will all go through times when it would be best for us to take a break from it altogether, or at least from certain types of incidents which might hit "too close to home." During all meetings and in-service trainings, members should be encouraged to feel free to communicate to their coordinators any changing life circumstance that might affect their performance. Keeping such confidential notes on their team roster makes it easier for a coordinator to pick members who are best suited to a situation or group. Brief notes might include "had SIDS death in family," "lost two parents in one year," "going through a nasty divorce," "was victim of crime," etc. Keeping such a list allows the coordinator to avoid putting a member in a difficult situation.

Some teams, in their selection of new members, make little attempt at the difficult task of excluding members based upon various selection criteria. As a result, it is not unusual for coordinators to designate some members for the performance of only specific or limited activities. For example, a member who exhibits poor boundaries by repeatedly telling personal stories during responses in spite of supervision may be limited to "sergeant-at-arms," or "administrative tasks only." Ideally, through supervision and guidance, a member would come to understand and agree to such limitations. But whether or not that is the case, such notes must be kept extremely confidential. See Appendices 5 and 6 for a sample of recordkeeping formats.

Quality Control

These are a group of activities which have relevance to the continued quality of a team's services and to the continued health and confidence of its members. As with the administrative, clinical, or recordkeeping functions, these quality control functions are not uniformly assigned to one role or person on the team. Some of these functions are commonly performed by the clinical director, some by team coordinators, some by others. Regardless of the person to whom they are assigned, regularly performing these functions can ensure the longevity and valued reputation of your team.

Outcome Assessment

At minimum, a post-service follow-up call should be made to the host or administrator of the organization served. It is often the on-call coordinator of a particular response who makes the first and last contact. The on-call coordinator begins by assessing needs and choosing services and ends with outcome assessment and follow-up. A sample of questions that a coordinator might ask are in Appendix 7.

Three or four simple questions can help evaluate the group's satisfaction, concerns, complaints, and need for more follow-up services. A sample of a satisfaction survey to be used by participants is included in Appendix 8. Bringing feedback from this contact back to your team might be a good piece of reinforcement. Conversely, if there *were* concerns or complaints about the team's activities, this may be an issue for supervision. It is very important to address any concerns of the organization that was served. Failing to either inquire about or respond to complaints often ensures that your services are not requested by an organization again.

Some teams have taken on a much more ambitious outcome assessment of methods and goals. One of the best examples in CISM literature is the seminal work of Ray Flannery (1998) who gathered and reported long-term data on changes in employee turnover rates, use of sick time, absenteeism, workman's compensation claims, and other objective measures of outcome. Performing almost any kind of outcome research can be a tremendous assistance to the organizations using these services, as well as to the CISM field as a whole.

Supervision

Supervision of team members is a quality control function, generally provided by a clinical director or a coordinator. Supervision is designed to provide team members a safe place to discuss their reactions to various professional challenges and to consolidate and learn from new experiences. When provided regularly in different settings and in comfortable surroundings, supervision can also be used to address more sensitive issues such as concerns about performance. Clinical supervision, whether in an individual or group format, is an essential support for CISM members and helps prevent burn-out or other deleterious effects.

The opportunity to supervise members in the development of skills is one of the main reasons for conducting role plays, table-tops, and other exercises. In most practice situations, the bulk of the supervision takes place in a group setting and comes as often from peers as from the clinical director or team coordinator. However, issues which are raised by strategically scripted role-play scenarios (e.g., anger, guilt, or grief) often are processed best in the privacy of a one-on-one supervision session. Providing this opportunity is a big part of the clinical director's job.

One of the purposes of supervision is to help members become aware of their own personal reactions to various material encountered in CISM work and to learn how to keep their reactions from getting in the way of the work. Creating opportunities for supervision is one of the main purposes of this guidebook. Want an individual to explore their own reactions to being openly challenged during a response? Try the "Challenging Comments Game." Want members to reflect on their own complex thought process during a response? Try a table-top exercise. Want to explore reactions to particular emotional themes? Turn to the "Facilitator's Guide Sheet" of any of the scenarios for a synopsis of prevalent themes therein.

Creating safe opportunities for supervision is part of the job of being a coordinator. Sometimes knowing a member's issues, strengths, and weaknesses is integral to the art of coordinating. For example, the knowledge (gained in supervision) that a member is a past victim of crime allows the coordinator to avoid a needlessly poor fit between that person and the current situation. Another time, it might be only in the safety of an individual supervision that a member processes a personal life crisis enough to place himself or herself on the inactive list. Both the team coordinator and the clinical director should make themselves available in different ways for individual supervision of members.

It has been mentioned earlier (see "Monitoring Team Performance") that teams should have a procedure by which members can request the supervision of another member. One format for this supervision is the debriefing of the debriefers, primarily because peers are helped to give constructive feedback or even criticism directly, hopefully thus maintaining enough mutual trust to continue working together. However, for many of the more thorny issues (ethical breach, repeated boundary violations, etc.) private supervision is the indicated format.

Providing supervision is part of both the science and the art of running a CISM team. It falls directly under a team coordinator's (and clinical director's) mission for the "care and feeding" of the team, as well as fulfilling monitoring and quality assurance functions.

SECTION 3

Continuing Education and Training

Even after team members have received their training and have some experience, their education should not end. Teams that are successful in maintaining their membership and services within the community often provide their members with on-going educational opportunities. This might include an annual training seminar for the team or shorter trainings at the regular team meetings.

These trainings work to keep the team skill levels up between calls, increase the skills of the team, and in general, keep them "fresh." It is probably not as important what is done, as that it is done on a regular basis. An exercise or two from this guidebook at quarterly meetings, with larger refresher trainings annually, is a reasonable expectation.

In deciding what to train, Raymond Flannery's research provides a refreshingly clear example of a logical premise: To help someone become more stress-resistant, identify and teach those skills used by the naturally "Stress-Resistant-Person" (Flannery, R.B. "Becoming Stress Resistant," 1994). Study those with natural skills, identify what they do, and teach others to do the same.

What are the skills of the best CISM workers? What goes through the mind of an experienced debriefer during a response? How can the coordinator or clinical director impart those things?

The **art of facilitating** involves training for:

- What one listens for
- What one thinks about and asks oneself
- How to remain focused in the presence of emotion and time demands

After all team members are familiar with the steps of the various responses and have a working understanding of the purposes of each phase and the basic mechanisms for making them work, additional training is required to assure the well-rounded competence of all team members. This training, as well as additional CISM, concentrates on listening skills that help the CISM team members uncover the underlying issues that will come up in each of the phases of the response. This also works when doing a one-on-one intervention.

While we have no interest in trying to make all team members into "mini mental health workers," we do think it is important that they work equally hard during each phase of the process. This includes listening intently during each phase to assure that by the teaching and re-entry phase, all of the major issues have been addressed.

Listening For Themes

We believe that in addition to teaching the steps necessary to do the various CISM responses, debriefers also need to learn to listen for the themes that generally emerge during an intervention.

We suggest that this can be accomplished by teaching the principles below while using the various scenarios that follow in the next section.

Each phase of an intervention brings forth information that is both factual (cognitive) and emotional (affective). When individuals are telling their story, it is important to listen for both. These themes are then used during the teaching and re-entry phases to make the education fit the needs of the individual or group receiving the service.

We encourage debriefers to follow the questions used during a debriefing as a method for organizing an intervention during a one-on-one session. By using empathic listening skills during the intervention, the debriefees will often disclose what is bothering them in the fashion that is described below—the same as would happen during a group.

Teaching people to listen for these themes when using the scenarios or games will enhance their abilities as debriefers. The following material underlies all teaching done to develop skilled debriefers.

Fact Phase (Debriefing)/Exploration Phase (Defusing)

The primary purpose of the fact/exploration phase is to equalize information among the participants, gain a complete understanding of the event in its many facets, and to begin to understand what parts of the event may be causing significant distress to the individual. As the group is answering the questions in the fact/exploration phase, the team should be listening for the following issues:

- Did any revealed fact contradict intake information?
- Did anyone reveal any factual information unknown to other debriefees?
- Was there any blaming going on regarding other debriefees or other groups?
- Based upon the information given, what are the significant factors that make this a critical incident for each individual? Who had "hands-on"? Who was more in the periphery?
- Is there enough information now for the group to understand the event?
- Were there any "surprise elements" to the story (i.e., personnel expecting one thing and finding something significantly different when they arrived)?

Thought Phase (Debriefing)/Exploration Phase (Defusing)

The primary purpose of the thought/exploration phase is to begin to lead the participants into a more introspective look at the effects of the event on themselves. Often, the thoughts that they have concerning the event reveal where they are most uncomfortable or feel guilty. As the group is answering the questions in the thought/exploration phase, the team should be listening for the following issues:

— Process themes:

- Did you pickup on any unrelated issues that one or more debriefees have?
- Did any debriefee link this event with previous events?
- Are there any similar thoughts from more than one debriefee that you can link and validate?

— Content themes (*Psychotraumatology*, Everly, 1988):

- Disruption of worldview as just or fair
- Abandonment or betrayal

- Violation of sense of self (self-esteem or worth)
- Destruction of sense of personal safety

Reaction Phase (Debriefing)

The primary purpose of the reaction phase is to allow participants to discuss their inner-most reactions to the event. This is usually the area in which they discuss how this event has been personalized by them, how the event has challenged their sense of personal safety, or attached concerns for members of their own family.

As the group is answering the questions in the reaction phase, the team should be listening for the following issues:

- Has this event slipped past their "protective shield" and been personalized by them?
- Did you sense that any debriefee is blocking this or other events?
- Did any debriefee appear to be making excuses to cover perceived self-guilt?
- What are the reactions that are common to more than one person in this group?
- Did you get any indication that the process frightened any debriefee?

Symptom Phase (Debriefing)

The primary goal of the symptom phase is to identify anything that the person has noticed that is different about themselves since the incident. The participants will struggle to give voice to their physical, emotional, cognitive, and behavioral struggles since the event.

- Did any debriefee indicate any symptoms that could be injurious (e.g., drinking and driving)?
- Did any debriefee appear to lack any kind of support system (no family or close friends)?
- What common reactions were not mentioned during the debriefing that you know have probably shown up (anger, guilt, etc.)?

Teaching Phase (Debriefing)/Information (Defusing)

The primary goal of the teaching/information phase is to highlight the major themes that the group has discussed during the debriefing and to do some practical teaching on those subjects. While the basic teaching concerning the issues of exercise, diet, and substance abuse should always be included, at times additional topics should be taught that are relevant to the specific issues of the group. Topics such as an understanding of the grief process, what to say to grieving family members, the protocols of the funeral, or the suicide thought processes, are especially helpful at times.

While one team member might have the primary responsibility of facilitating the teaching phase, the team should be listening for the following issues:

- What were the major themes you heard?
- Were they covered by the facilitator of this phase?
- What do you want to add or emphasize as part of this phase?

Training Strategies

In this section we describe five teaching strategies for providing training within the team. The first is the use of **One-on-One Role Plays**, the second is **Table-Top Exercises**, the third is the use of **Small Group Role Plays**, the fourth is the use of **Group Exercises**, and the last is some **Games** a team might play.

These strategies were developed mainly for training in the following CISM components:

- Individual (one-on-one interventions)
- Defusings
- Debriefings (CISD)
- Crisis Management Briefings (CMB)

While many of the scenarios set up situations ripe for a CMB, the scripts are tailored to create realistic group interactions, and any single page of script from any scenario could provide enough background for the practice of one-on-one crisis intervention, and at least discussion material for the other interventions.

One-on-One Role Plays

Role of the Educational Facilitator

In the one-on-one exercise, the facilitator is responsible for setting the stage for a dynamic, positive experience for the students. As a one-on-one debriefer you need to learn as much as possible about how this person is viewing and reacting to the recent event. Many individuals may have participated in similar exercises in previous training and may be reluctant to engage in this activity.

The importance of debriefers having good listening skills cannot be overstated. When the communication is between only two individuals (debriefee and debriefer), the debriefer needs to read and interpret the body language and what the debriefee is saying or not saying in order to provide meaningful feedback and observations.

Getting Organized

First, the educational facilitator **chooses the roles** from the scenarios in Section 4 he/she is going to use for the one-on-one activity. The facilitator should pay particular attention to the potential issues that arise based upon the information provided in the scenario. In this exercise there are three roles: a **Speaker**, a **Listener**, and an **Observer**. The educational facilitator counts the number of participants, divides this number by three (as there will be three roles) to determine the total number of triads, and has the students count off from one to the total number (i.e., 30 in the group divided by three equals ten, so you have them count off by ten). Your instructions at this point are: all the "1's" get together here, the "2's" get together, etc. By counting off in larger numbers you will often break up friends into different groups. This also encourages building new team relationships among the participants.

The **participants are now divided** into these groups of three. The educational facilitator arranges the groups in different parts of the room with two individuals (speaker and listener) facing each other and the third (observer) seated to the side.
The educational facilitator asks the **participants to introduce themselves**, particularly if there is anyone who might be new to the group.

Getting Volunteers

The participants will play each of the three roles (speaker, listener, and observer) in this exercise, which will enable them to appreciate the particular issues each faces. With each rotation a different role from one of the scenarios will be used.

Instructions to the Groups

At this point the facilitator will **give directions to the entire group**. The groups will select one speaker, one listener, and one observer. The speaker will be given one of the exercises from one of the scenarios in Section 4. The speaker will then assume this role and tell his/her experience to the listener. The listener will demonstrate his/her ability to appropriately draw out the speaker, observe his/her body language, ask questions, and provide appropriate feedback. The observer will remain silent throughout the exercise and will note strengths and weaknesses on the part of the listener for later discussion. After approximately 15 minutes (the educational facilitator may vary this time period), the exercise will conclude and the three individuals will discuss how well the listener was able to interpret the speaker and provide the speaker with meaningful and supportive comments. At the direction of the educational facilitator, the groups will then rotate the speaker, listener, and observer roles, be given another role, and repeat the process.

Frequently, there is a tendency for listeners to provide a repetitive feedback statement such as "What I hear you saying is...." Participants should be encouraged to avoid using repetitious devices such as these because they can be interpreted as too rote.

It is beneficial to provide an opportunity for the entire **group to share their experiences** with the rest of the group after all rotations have been completed. Three copies of the "Observers Feedback Form" (Appendix 9) should be provided to each triad as a guideline for processing the experience.

Getting Started

The educational facilitator asks the speakers to read quietly through the scenario, his/her role, and issues that are identified in the **Thought**, **Reaction**, and **Symptom** sections of the scenario.

It is important that all groups start each round at the same time and finish when directed to do so by the facilitator. During this exercise the educational facilitator moves around the room, listening in on the groups.

After each person has participated in each of the three positions, the educational facilitator moderates a discussion of the activity. The facilitator should allow for the free exchange of ideas among the participants and only move on when the material becomes repetitive.

Processing the Experience

Questions such as the following are used to trigger meaningful discussions:

- "What did you hear that you will try to remember for your own use?"
- "What part of the process did you find most important?"
- "What part might have been the most challenging for you?"
- "What was the most helpful statement made by the listener?"
- "What statement might have been more helpful?"

Table-Top Exercises

Table-top exercises use the same scenarios as the role plays. The major difference is that in a table-top exercise, all the participants have the opportunity to share their thoughts, expertise, comments, and assessments after each individual in the scenario and after each phase in the intervention. Table-top exercises do not involve actually practicing the skills, but rely on a more cognitive approach to learning. They take some of the "pressure to perform" away and are more of a relaxed group effort.

Role of the Educational Facilitator

The facilitator is responsible for making this a fun, educational, and positive experience for all involved. This task sounds more daunting than it actually is. People who are attracted to doing this type of work are usually willing to be nice to one another. They are interested in learning the model and being helpful to each other, so the process usually goes very well.

If you are enthusiastic and positive in your approach, the participants will follow your lead. The most challenging task for the educational facilitator is to make sure that all feedback is presented in a positive manner. No matter how poorly someone might have done, it is your responsibility to turn it into a positive learning experience. For example, "I bet you will never forget to do that again" or "Thanks for giving us a great example of how things can sometimes go wrong and giving your team members an opportunity to practice working out of it." Of course, it is also true that by doing these training scenarios you will sometimes learn that someone is ill-suited to doing crisis response work. There are many roles on a CISM team besides frontline work that people can do and still be a part of the team. Learning that in practice is better than learning it in real life.

Getting Organized

First, the educational facilitator **chooses the scenario** he/she is going to use for the table-top simulation. The facilitator should pay particular attention to the potential issues that arise based upon the information provided in the scenario.

Next, the facilitator decides which of the interventions is going to be practiced. If a **One-on-One** is being practiced, a single page of any scenario is chosen and the group as a whole discusses the "victim's" likely issues and the intervener's possible questions and prompts.

If a **Defusing or CISD** is chosen, the group discussion is a "walk-through" of each stage of the respective response, often character by character.

If a **Crisis Management Briefing** is chosen, the group simply discusses the issues they might expect to emerge in each phase of the briefing.

The table-top process works better if all the **participants are seated in a circle** similar to an intervention. This room arrangement encourages participant interactions.

The educational facilitator asks all the **participants to introduce themselves**, particularly if there is anyone who might be new to the group.

As previously noted, there is a tendency for the facilitator to lead the participants during the discussion phases. To avoid this, the facilitator should restrict his/her comments to statements that reflect or summarize the participants' statements (i.e., "Then, you anticipate that may be an issue for one of the individuals in the scenario?"). The facilitator can also ask if any of the other participants also picked up on this and what specifically suggested this as an issue. Participants should be allowed to share their thoughts on any of the issues suggested.

Getting Volunteers

A nice part of using a table-top simulation is that **everyone "volunteers."** The discussion allows all trainees to have input and ideas about what the participants might be experiencing in each of the phases. The educational facilitator moderates the discussions, encourages novice debriefers, and tactfully prevents individuals from monopolizing the discussion.

Instructions to the Team

The facilitator explains that he/she will **read the incident statement** of the selected scenario and the list of personnel involved. Participants listen to what is read and any other information that may be suggested by the roles of the debriefees. The educational facilitator provides the opportunity for the participants to ask for any clarification of what has been read. He/she then asks a question such as, **"What issues do you anticipate in this intervention?"** or **"Does anyone on the list of personnel involved suggest a problem issue for the group?"**

The facilitator should allow for the free exchange of ideas among the participants and only move on to the next phase when the material becomes repetitive.

The table-top simulation works best if allowed to develop at its own pace. Occasionally, more experienced debriefers may inadvertently restrict or limit the discussion by pronouncements such as: "The major issue of this intervention is..." or "That person is probably going to have to deal with ...." The skillful facilitator attempts to draw out the clues which suggested the observation and give other participants an opportunity to ask the veteran what he/she picked up on to arrive at this conclusion.

Getting Started

The educational facilitator **reads the synopsis of the incident aloud** and asks if there are any questions. Once he/she is sure that everyone understands the situation being portrayed, the facilitator **reads each person's role in the incident**. The participants are then asked to **anticipate the issues that may be facing each of the group members** (i.e., guilt, anger, etc.).

This process is **repeated for each of the phases** of the technique being practiced. During this period, the educational facilitator refrains from confirming or denying any of the issues suggested by the participants. Frequently, experienced debriefers are able to pick up critical information from the incident information and the roles of the debriefees. Less-experienced debriefers often glean this skill from listening to their colleagues.

For example, in a scenario regarding the death of a young child, the experienced debriefer considers the possibility that the participants may have children the same age as the victim(s). This awareness allows the debriefer to be on the alert to this as a potential issue during the subsequent phases. Sometimes this knowledge can assist the debriefer in drawing out issues the participants might be trying to avoid.

The fact phase, in addition to reassuring the debriefees that they are in a safe environment, is how the debriefees view their role in the event. Often individuals will downplay their role with statements such as: "I just did my job" or "that is what they hire us to do." During the discussion following the fact phase, participants start to hone-in more precisely on the issues.

In the thought phase, participants start demonstrating issues that make their experience of this event unlike similar events to them. In the discussion, the facilitator needs to allow the participants the opportunity to express insights they have picked up during this phase.

In the reaction phase, individuals are the most vulnerable because it is here they are sharing their deepest emotions with their colleagues. Debriefers need to exercise all of their listening skills in this phase because it may be what is not said that is significant. The participants should discuss both the expressed and silent issues. It is here that debriefers can start to comment on how the debriefees are processing the event.

The symptom phase often expresses the immediate impairments debriefees are having in the processing of the event. This is a significant time for the debriefees and they should not be rushed through this phase. The educational facilitator can direct a discussion on ways participants can honor these concerns during a debriefing.

Because the teaching and re-entry phases do not provide input from the debriefees, the educational facilitator asks the participants to focus on what to include in both of these phases. This discussion can provide all the participants with powerful techniques that will assist the debriefees in viewing their reactions as normal reactions of normal people to an abnormal event.

Processing The Experience

Questions such as the following are used to trigger meaningful discussions:

- "What did you hear that you'll try to remember for your own use?"
- "What part of the process did you find most important?"
- "What part might have been the most challenging for you?"

Small Group Role Plays

A CISM associate from Texas once said about role play, "It's a lot harder ropin' that calf when it's runnin', isn't it?" We're pretty sure he was referring to the unique demand characteristics of role-play practice—that one must practice in front of others and in real-time, not to mention the fact that role play can sometimes bring out the ham in people who can't resist spicing things up a bit with a display of emotion. When asked for a clarification, we believe our Texan friend affirmed this interpretation when he added that, "It's harder comin' up with slick soundin' things to say when you're jugglin' on stage."

Role play attempts to add some realistic emotional demands to the practice situation. The circle of faces waiting to hear what you'll say and the number of things you're thinking about (jugglin') while trying to appear focused (be respectful, look smart, get them talking to each other, act confident, this person's anger, that person's grief) all add up to a taste of the real thing. A good role-play is experiential learning at its best. Most trainers are quite familiar with the paradox that the same participants who practically hid under the table to avoid being in a role play are the same ones who later praise the experience as the most valuable of the whole workshop when they fill out their evaluation and wonder why you didn't provide more of them.

The following training sequence makes sense for learning any of the ten CISM techniques:

- Read about and memorize the model
- Watch two examples
- Practice specific skills or building blocks (introductions, table-top, etc.)
- Role play two examples
- Attend two real responses as back-up
- Facilitate a response

No one can learn how to conduct an ICISF model debriefing or defusing by only going to a workshop, reading about them in books, watching videotapes, or watching other people do them. It is only after doing all of the above, and by sitting in a group and actually doing the work, that one actually learns how to do it by actually doing it.

In some cases, this may consist of "on the job" learning by participating in defusings or debriefings with more experienced team members. Actually, all of us learn this way every time we go into the field and do our work. Even the most experienced debriefing personnel can learn something new or be reminded of techniques during an actual defusing or debriefing.

Getting Organized

To begin, the educational facilitator must decide what he/she is attempting to accomplish with the experience. Is it to teach only the rookies? Is it to provide experience for all members present? How many experienced team members are present to assist? The answers to these types of questions will determine if you are going to have one group operating with everyone else observing, or have multiple groups operating at the same time. This decision has several ramifications depending upon the purposes of the educational facilitator.

The advantages of having one group with everyone else observing is that the educational material is consistent. That is, everyone sees the same debriefing and during the processing of the experience, hears common issues discussed. The facilitator remains in control of the entire process and there is little risk of a bad example being set forth as a model. This method is often used when demonstrating the model for the first time or when trying to maximize the common experience.

The disadvantages of using only one group with observers is that only a small number of individuals get to practice their skills and the group process is sometimes more inhibited because of the observers.

The advantages of dividing the entire group into simultaneous debriefing sessions are that everyone participates and experiences the debriefing process, more people get to practice their skills, and you limit the "fishbowl" experience of being observed by an audience. It's often fun to see how two identical scenarios sometimes result in completely different discussions.

The disadvantages of having several groups going at once is that more facilitators are needed, since it is unwise to conduct a role play without someone observing the group. The processing of the group experience is therefore more challenging. Other coordinators or experienced members are often pressed into service to supervise.

If a **CISD or defusing** is being practiced, assign all roles of a scenario to a group of volunteers, and identify a CISM team to go through the requisite number of stages for the response.

If a **CMB** is being practiced, a scenario is chosen and a volunteer CISM team addresses the rest of the audience as to the facts of the incident and fields their questions

Once the **CISM teams are identified**, they are given a copy of the role sheet and **sent out of the room with instructions to organize themselves**, i.e., pick a facilitator, divide introductory comments, etc.

Another technique is to **send a "host" from the affected agency out to answer any questions** the team might have. This simulates actually arriving at the facility and doing their last minute check of the current situation. Often, new facts are learned and this step in the procedure is reinforced. Some of the scenarios provide opportunities for the team to make decisions about the personnel who are present for the debriefing, but who may not be appropriate, at least at first glance. The "host/hostess" is instructed to give the basic information provided, but not to volunteer too much information unless specifically prompted by a question from the team.

If the debriefing team fails to ask enough questions they may find themselves surprised during the exercise. This can be a part of the learning experience. During the processing of the event, the educational facilitator can make use of the example and provide some information about good questions to ask before entering the room

Getting Volunteers

Be creative in getting the volunteers necessary to do the exercise. Briefly explain what the critical incident is and tell people that if it is too close to an incident of their own they have the option of sitting out of this experience, perhaps serving as process observers.

It is sometimes beneficial for natural groups to form. At other times, it is best to mix up the group so that they get to experience working with people with whom they might not ordinarily come into contact. The important part of this is to simply decide beforehand and quickly move the group into their configurations.

If using one group, then **ask for volunteers and have them move into a circle**. It is often true that asking for volunteers just before a break, and indicating that the break is contingent upon getting them, speeds up the process. The more people "volunteer" the better they feel, although if done with humor, most folks involve themselves willingly. **Then ask for three volunteers within the group to serve as debriefers**.

Instructions to the Participants

The educational facilitator gets the groups organized into circles and makes sure there are enough chairs available in the circle for the CISM team as well as the group members. The **individual roles for the experience are distributed** at this time and people are given an opportunity to review them. It is a good idea to have the **participants identify to each other the role they play within the scenario** ("I am the victim's best friend," "I was first on scene," etc.), because several members of the group will have interacted during the event and it is helpful to know who did what.

Once the group understands their roles, it is important that other instructions are given. To make this a positive learning experience, role players should be urged to **"Imagine *yourself* in this situation, how would you react?"** Further cautions such as, **"Don't overplay your role or be the worst person you can imagine in a debriefing,"** are generally given. Consider light-heartedly telling them that if they wish to portray this type of person, they will be the "lone debriefer" in the last role play of the training and everyone in their group will be allowed to act out. Role play is more about *presenting* thoughts and reactions than acting them out. These cautions establish the ground rules for the experience and usually lead to a fairly realistic portrayal of the aftermath of an incident.

> Collect all role-play script sheets before beginning because people tend to read from them or play with them throughout the exercise.

Other favorite instructions are:

- No worst-case scenarios
- Don't "ham it up" or overact your part
- Keep it brief
- Remember to act as if you were actually friends

Instructions to the Host/Hostess

It should not be anyone's intent to deceive the debriefing team. *However,* sometimes we do not have all the information we might have needed before going in to do our work. Therefore, the instructions are basically to **stick with the facts** of the situation and to **answer the questions that the team asks**. Sometimes the team may fail to ask a critical question like, "Is there any blaming going on?" **Try not to volunteer too much information**, but do try to cover the basics of the situation and **identify your personnel who are waiting for the team**.

Some of the role plays have members that perhaps should not be in the debriefing. Perhaps they were not on scene, are not part of the agency, or for some other reason might not fit. The key factor here is for the team to discover it and make a choice on whether to include or exclude the individual and determine how they are going to do it. This is a good discussion point after the role-play is finished.

If you do not elect to have a host/hostess, the educational facilitator should play this role.

Instructions to the Audience

To assure the minimum disruption to the group process, if there are people not directly participating in the exercise it is good to tell them to remain quiet and **to move close enough to be able to hear**. It is their responsibility to get close enough, not the group's responsibility to talk louder. They might also be asked to pay special attention to some part of the experience such as the body language, voice tones, and things that the team did that made the experience helpful. The CISD Observation Sheet in Appendix 10 is excellent for this purpose.

The audience is told to **hold their questions and comments** until after the experience is finished and the debriefees and debriefers have had an opportunity to discuss their common experience.

Instructions to the Process Observers (Optional)

Sometimes you may wish to assign experienced personnel to the role of **Process Observer**. Their responsibility is to pay attention to the overall process of the group, watching for things that the team did well, things that might have been done differently, or where things might have taken a wrong turn. The process observers are especially helpful if you are doing multiple groups at once, since the educational facilitator cannot be in all places at the same time.

Process observers then assume the same responsibility that the educational facilitator has of making the experience a positive one. They should be focused on what went well, what was helpful, and keep a positive discussion on what might not have gone so well. It would be helpful to use the CISD Observation Sheet in Appendix 10.

What Happens Next?

Sometimes this is the hardest part for the educational facilitator, because you must just **let the process unfold.** You are not a member of the debriefing/defusing team, so you are invisible, and should not answer questions once the role play begins. If the team gets into trouble, let them find their way out of it. After all, you would not be there in a real-life situation. People will often learn more after a difficult experience and usually not repeat their mistakes. If the team gets really lost for a long time, or the session turns ugly, you can of course interrupt it for guidance or redirection.

Most of the simulations in this workbook will take about 45 minutes to complete. If they begin to run a little long, in the interest of time you can step in and say something like "I am taking a slice of time here, let's say that you have now finished this phase and are ready to move into the next one." This sometimes occurs during the reaction phase.

Processing the Experience

Depending upon the number of groups that have been working on this exercise, processing the experience is usually pretty straightforward. Ask the debriefees to move back a little and bring the debriefers into a tight circle in the middle of the debriefees. Use the debriefing the debriefers model to **help the CISM team review its performance**—what worked and what did not—always offering them positive alternatives. For example, if someone asked an inappropriate question, one might ask, "What were you attempting to accomplish? How else could that have been done?" Utilizing feedback from the other debriefers during this process is also a very good idea.

Once the debriefing of the debriefers is finished**, ask the participants for input**. How do they think it went? What did the team members do that "felt good" or made the process go well? It is usually a good idea not to focus on what went wrong once you leave the debriefers circle. As the educational facilitator, your job is to make this as positive a learning experience as you can.

When the participants are finished, **ask observers outside the circle** for their observations and questions. **Focus on things they liked** and will try to remember as models for their own work.

The concluding activity is to ask the participants to share their thoughts on how the intervention went, what they learned from their fellow participants, any issues they might have personalized, and how they are going to take care of themselves after this exercise. For a more complete review, refer to "Debriefing the Debriefers" in Section 2.

SECTION 4

Practice Scenarios

Introduction

The following sections contain role-play scenarios that simulate a variety of situations that a team is likely to encounter during the course of their work. They are grouped by the population targeted for intervention.

In each sub-section, you will find two scenarios that are a variation of the same event. This is done for two reasons. The first is that many educational facilitators might want to merely open the guidebook to this section and copy a role play for use. Thus, having the "car crash" and "staff suicide" in each section allows the reader quick access to this type of situation.

The second reason is to show the reader that, with minor changes, many of the different scenarios can be altered to meet a specific population that you might be training.

While there is only one complete scenario printed in each sub-section of this book, the files on the Sub-Section Summary page are complete files (one page for every participant in each scenario) on the CD-ROM. We intend that the CD-ROM is the easiest method for printing a role play scenario.

For training purposes only, scenarios can be photocopied from this guidebook or printed from the .PDF files included on the accompanying CD-ROM.

Writing Your Own Scenarios

Most scenarios are based on real-life events that have been experienced in past interventions. It is important to record your thoughts as soon as possible after the defusing or debriefing so that you can capture the issues that developed. It is also essential that you change enough information to make identification with the real-life event impossible.

When you return from an intervention that has a significant component that you want to capture, jot down notes to yourself indicating the issues, the role of the participants (without any names) and their contributions to the process, and any other items that affected the intervention. Next, change locations, offices, services, individuals (if the real-life event has a 30-year-old male you might change him to a 50-year-old female without changing any of the input), and basic facts about the event (if the individual was stabbed to death, you might have him die by gunshot wounds). This process assures that anyone who was present in the intervention would not recognize the individuals or event. Sometimes you can combine two or three interventions into your new creative scenario without changing the issues that you want to use as a teaching tool.

It is best to use a standard format for writing the scenarios. A Word template for writing your own scenarios is included on the CD-ROM (ScenarioTemplate.doc).

Develop an overview sheet and a role sheet for each participant in the scenario. In "The Incident" box, describe the scenario. In the "Your Role In This Event" space, provide the significance of this participant in the scenario. Sometimes individuals are added to provide roles for larger groups in role plays (i.e., you can always add an additional firefighter or police officer in EMS scenarios or another teacher or office worker in community scenarios).

In the space provided for each of the phases, try to provide information in one or two sentences that will allow the significance of the role to come through. Experience has shown that in role plays, individuals tend to add information (it is generally advisable to caution participants in role plays to restrict their improvisations).

Once you have finished writing the scenario, ask a colleague to review it for consistency and realism. Note any appropriate corrections each time you use the scenario in training and update your saved file.

Scenarios A.1 - A.13

FIREFIGHTER-BASED EXPERIENCES

Scenario A.1
Double Fatality (Multi-Incident Experience)

Scenario A.2
Firefighter Car Crash

Scenario A.3
Multi-Fatility House Fire

Scenario A.4
Teenager Car Crash

Scenario A.5
Teenage Overdose

Scenario A.6
Firefighter Suicide

Scenario A.7
Fire Chief's Son

Scenario A.8
Single Fatality Accident

Scenario A.9
Ambulance Crash

Scenario A.10
Fire Fatalities

Scenario A.11
Firefighter Injury

Scenario A.12
Aerial Platform Collapse

Scenario A.13
Firefighter Sudden Impact

Scenario A.1

Double Fatality

Facilitator's Guide Sheet

THE INCIDENT:

The Central Township Fire Department responded to a car-tree collision in a rural part of the county. When they arrived on scene, they found that both the driver and passenger were dead. The driver was an 85-year old male and the passenger was his 82-year old wife.

The location of the accident was approximately 400 yards east of a blinking yellow/red traffic controlled intersection that frequently has accidents due to the speed on the north-south (yellow flashing light) highway. ***In fact, this same department had been dispatched to this same intersection about three months ago when a family of four had been killed.***

The engine arrived on scene first with the two firefighters. Two volunteer firefighters arrived within five minutes, shortly before the ambulance. The paramedic received permission from medical control for a dead-on-scene call for the two victims. It was necessary to use the Jaws of Life to remove both bodies, as it was a head-on crash into the tree.

It took approximately 20 minutes to extricate the two bodies, which were transported in body bags to the local hospital morgue. The total time out on scene was about one hour and thirty minutes. The victims were residents of the township and two of the firefighters thought that they knew who they were, but didn't know either very well.

PLACE: Central Township

TIME: One week ago: 9:45 p.m.

PERSONNEL INVOLVED:	MAJOR ISSUE:	SYMPTOMS:
1. Fire chief	Probably does not belong in group	
2. Incident commander	Reactions from previous	Nightmares; overprotective
3. Second firefighter	Reactions from previous	Intrusive images
4. First volunteer firefighter	Memories from previous	Sleep problems; avoidance
5. Second volunteer firefighter	Memories from previous	Thinking of quitting
6. First paramedic	None	None
7. Second paramedic	Memories from previous	Anxious; overprotective

POSSIBLE PROCESS QUESTIONS:

- How was the issue of the chief being included/excluded handled?
- Would you do anything different in the future?
- Was it a good call to have this debriefing?
- Can this response, after so long, help mitigate the effects of the previous incident?
- What symptoms were shared that may have been kept secret for months?

Scenario A.1

Double Fatality

Overview

THE INCIDENT:

The Central Township Fire Department responded to a car-tree collision in a rural part of the county. When they arrived on scene, they found that both the driver and passenger were dead. The driver was an 85-year old male and the passenger was his 82-year old wife.

The location of the accident was approximately 400 yards east of a blinking yellow/red traffic controlled intersection that frequently has accidents due to the speed on the north-south (yellow flashing light) highway. ***In fact, this same department had been dispatched to this same intersection about three months ago when a family of four had been killed.***

The engine arrived on scene first with the two firefighters. Two volunteer firefighters arrived within five minutes, shortly before the ambulance. The paramedic received permission from medical control for a dead-on-scene call for the two victims. It was necessary to use the Jaws of Life to remove both bodies, as it was a head-on crash into the tree.

It took approximately 20 minutes to extricate the two bodies, which were transported in body bags to the local hospital morgue. The total time out on scene was about one hour and thirty minutes. The victims were residents of the township and two of the firefighters thought that they knew who they were, but didn't know either very well.

PLACE: Central Township

TIME: One week ago: 9:45 p.m.

PERSONNEL INVOLVED:

1. Fire chief
2. Incident commander
3. Second firefighter
4. First volunteer firefighter
5. Second volunteer firefighter
6. First paramedic
7. Second paramedic

Scenario A.1

Double Fatality

Fire Chief

THE INCIDENT:

The Central Township Fire Department responded to a car-tree collision in a rural part of the county. When they arrived on scene, they found that both the driver and passenger were dead. The driver was an 85-year old male and the passenger was his 82-year old wife.

The location of the accident was approximately 400 yards east of a blinking yellow/red traffic controlled intersection that frequently has accidents due to the speed on the north-south (yellow flashing light) highway. ***In fact, this same department had been dispatched to this same intersection about three months ago when a family of four had been killed.***

The engine arrived on scene first with the two firefighters. Two volunteer firefighters arrived within five minutes, shortly before the ambulance. The paramedic received permission from medical control for a dead-on-scene call for the two victims. It was necessary to use the Jaws of Life to remove both bodies, as it was a head-on crash into the tree.

It took approximately 20 minutes to extricate the two bodies, which were transported in body bags to the local hospital morgue. The total time out on scene was about one hour and thirty minutes. The victims were residents of the township and two of the firefighters thought that they knew who they were, but didn't know either very well.

YOUR ROLE IN THIS INCIDENT:

The department is suburban-to-rural and adjacent to a major city. The township-wide department is divided into three zones. Each zone has a fire station that is manned 24/7 by two firefighters. The fire chief has an on-call assistant chief in each of the three zones.

In addition, volunteers who are paid on-call firefighters respond to calls in their zone. Five years ago, all of the paid and volunteer firefighters went though medical first responder training and the department responds to medical emergencies as well as fire calls.

One of your assistant chiefs indicated to you that one of the zones had a double fatality last Friday evening. Since then, the assistant fire chief has noticed a change in attitudes on the part of both the paid and on-call staff.

As fire chief, you recently attended a countywide chiefs association meeting where you heard about CISM interventions. You are inquiring if this service is available and the cost of the service. You can arrange to use the boardroom at the township hall to do the debriefing. You will also approve pay for all the full-time and on-call firefighters from zone three. You will have zone three covered by the assistant chief for that zone during the debriefing. Neither you nor the assistant chief was on scene.

You are aware that an accident had occurred near this same site about three months ago and a family was killed, including two children. You know some of your personnel responded to it, but since you were not there, you don't know many of the details.

Scenario A.1

Double Fatality

First Firefighter / Incident Commander

THE INCIDENT:

The Central Township Fire Department responded to a car-tree collision in a rural part of the county. When they arrived on scene, they found that both the driver and passenger were dead. The driver was an 85-year old male and the passenger was his 82-year old wife.

The location of the accident was approximately 400 yards east of a blinking yellow/red traffic controlled intersection that frequently has accidents due to the speed on the north-south (yellow flashing light) highway. ***In fact, this same department had been dispatched to this same intersection about three months ago when a family of four had been killed.***

The engine arrived on scene first with the two firefighters. Two volunteer firefighters arrived within five minutes, shortly before the ambulance. The paramedic received permission from medical control for a dead-on-scene call for the two victims. It was necessary to use the Jaws of Life to remove both bodies, as it was a head-on crash into the tree.

It took approximately 20 minutes to extricate the two bodies, which were transported in body bags to the local hospital morgue. The total time out on scene was about one hour and thirty minutes. The victims were residents of the township and two of the firefighters thought that they knew who they were, but didn't know either very well.

YOUR ROLE IN THIS INCIDENT:

You are one of the full-time firefighters from zone three. You drove the engine to the scene of the accident. Your partner was initially responsible for assessing the two victims.

In the fact phase, share any of the information provided above.

In the thought phase, share the following information: The first thought that came into your mind when you received the call was that this was a short distance down the road from the controlled intersection where an entire family had been killed in a car accident three months and two days ago.

In the reaction phase, share the following information: You can't figure out why the department is holding this session for this accident. The accident there three months and two days ago was a real nightmare that still bothers you. At the previous accident, you and your partner had trouble locating the victims because of the amount of damage to the vehicle. You remember particularly how you first saw only the child's shoe under the rubble in the back seat. You reached to pick it up and found it attached to the leg of a child who was the same age as your daughter. You still remember the look on the child's face when you removed her from the wreckage. She looked just like she was asleep at night. That evening you woke your daughter several times just to make sure that she was still alive.

In the symptom phase, share the following information: You have been having nightmares about the previous accident. You have become over-protective of your daughter. You have been angry with your wife about taking your daughter with her too much in the car.

Scenario A.1

Double Fatality

Second Firefighter

THE INCIDENT:

The Central Township Fire Department responded to a car-tree collision in a rural part of the county. When they arrived on scene, they found that both the driver and passenger were dead. The driver was an 85-year old male and the passenger was his 82-year old wife.

The location of the accident was approximately 400 yards east of a blinking yellow/red traffic controlled intersection that frequently has accidents due to the speed on the north-south (yellow flashing light) highway. ***In fact, this same department had been dispatched to this same intersection about three months ago when a family of four had been killed.***

The engine arrived on scene first with the two firefighters. Two volunteer firefighters arrived within five minutes, shortly before the ambulance. The paramedic received permission from medical control for a dead-on-scene call for the two victims. It was necessary to use the Jaws of Life to remove both bodies, as it was a head-on crash into the tree.

It took approximately 20 minutes to extricate the two bodies, which were transported in body bags to the local hospital morgue. The total time out on scene was about one hour and thirty minutes. The victims were residents of the township and two of the firefighters thought that they knew who they were, but didn't know either very well.

YOUR ROLE IN THIS INCIDENT:

You immediately gained access to the vehicle and determined that neither victim was breathing or had a pulse. Due to the massive injuries, their age, and the fact that both victims were entangled in the car, you did not start CPR. You then helped stabilize the car for extrication.

In the fact phase, share any of the information provided above.

In the thought phase, share the following information: You remember this intersection because you have to cross from west to east on the flashing red light. You were also on the call three months and two days ago and remember the chaos.

In the reaction phase, share the following information: There isn't a day that goes by that you don't think about the accident in which the whole family was killed. You are glad that you don't have children at this point because you see how your friends have been having problems with child victims. In addition, the previous accident involved a gasoline spill that put more pressure on the firefighters. You also remember how the police officer left his siren running though the entire extrication. You can close your eyes and see the whole surreal scene.

In the symptom phase, share the following information: You had always thought that you could leave the job at the station, but you have discovered that when you least expect it, the scene can flash in front of your eyes whenever anyone mentions the accident. It was real hard with your friends who wanted to hear all the gory details after that accident. You can't understand why anyone would want to look at pictures of the accident in the newspaper, see it on the television news, or hear about it from someone who was on scene.

Scenario A.1

Double Fatality

First Volunteer Firefighter

THE INCIDENT:

The Central Township Fire Department responded to a car-tree collision in a rural part of the county. When they arrived on scene, they found that both the driver and passenger were dead. The driver was an 85-year old male and the passenger was his 82-year old wife.

The location of the accident was approximately 400 yards east of a blinking yellow/red traffic controlled intersection that frequently has accidents due to the speed on the north-south (yellow flashing light) highway. ***In fact, this same department had been dispatched to this same intersection about three months ago when a family of four had been killed.***

The engine arrived on scene first with the two firefighters. Two volunteer firefighters arrived within five minutes, shortly before the ambulance. The paramedic received permission from medical control for a dead-on-scene call for the two victims. It was necessary to use the Jaws of Life to remove both bodies, as it was a head-on crash into the tree.

It took approximately 20 minutes to extricate the two bodies, which were transported in body bags to the local hospital morgue. The total time out on scene was about one hour and thirty minutes. The victims were residents of the township and two of the firefighters thought that they knew who they were, but didn't know either very well.

YOUR ROLE IN THIS INCIDENT:

You were the first volunteer to arrive on scene. The incident commander sent you back to the intersection to divert traffic from the area. You parked your vehicle sideways in the road with the flashing lights on and stood near the intersection directing all eastbound traffic either north or south. As soon as the sheriff's deputy relieved you, you returned to assist with extrication.

In the fact phase, share any of the information provided above.

In the thought phase, share the following information: Your first thought concerned the fast traffic on the north-south road at the controlled intersection. You have been to five or six accidents at this intersection in the last three years.

In the reaction phase, share the following information: This scene reminded you of the accident three months and two days ago. You remember the news media at that earlier accident. One of the cameramen actually got in the way of firefighters. That scene was an unbelievable cluster with all the EMS vehicles, police cars, and spectators milling around. You even noticed one person smoking a cigarette despite the fact there was a large gasoline spill.

In the symptom phase, share the following information: Probably the nightmares are the worst thing you remember. You can't watch news programs anymore. You can't watch the TV programs "ER," "Emergency," or "COPS" because they bring back memories of that accident. Your wife enjoys those programs and gets upset when you leave the room as soon as they come on the television.

Scenario A.1

Double Fatality

Second Volunteer Firefighter

THE INCIDENT:

The Central Township Fire Department responded to a car-tree collision in a rural part of the county. When they arrived on scene, they found that both the driver and passenger were dead. The driver was an 85-year old male and the passenger was his 82-year old wife.

The location of the accident was approximately 400 yards east of a blinking yellow/red traffic controlled intersection that frequently has accidents due to the speed on the north-south (yellow flashing light) highway. ***In fact, this same department had been dispatched to this same intersection about three months ago when a family of four had been killed.***

The engine arrived on scene first with the two firefighters. Two volunteer firefighters arrived within five minutes, shortly before the ambulance. The paramedic received permission from medical control for a dead-on-scene call for the two victims. It was necessary to use the Jaws of Life to remove both bodies, as it was a head-on crash into the tree.

It took approximately 20 minutes to extricate the two bodies, which were transported in body bags to the local hospital morgue. The total time out on scene was about one hour and thirty minutes. The victims were residents of the township and two of the firefighters thought that they knew who they were, but didn't know either very well.

YOUR ROLE IN THIS INCIDENT:

You arrived just behind the first volunteer. The incident commander had you turn the westbound traffic around. You were relieved shortly by a sheriff's deputy and returned to assist with extrication. You were on the previous accident three month ago.

In the fact phase, share any of the information provided above.

In the thought phase, share the following information: When you received the page, your first thought was that there was another accident at bloody corners. All of the firefighters in the township know that half of all the major auto accidents have been at this intersection. You were on the scene three months ago when there were four fatalities.

In the reaction phase, share the following information: At the four-person fatality accident you were responsible for fire suppression. There was gasoline all over the place and spectators were actually walking in it. You also remember seeing one spectator discard a lighted cigarette near the gasoline spill. Everyone in the department has avoided talking about that accident because of the memories. You all took medical training so that you could help save lives, yet there was nothing you could do that night.

In the symptom phase, share the following information: You have thought about quitting as a volunteer firefighter. While you have always enjoyed the friendship of your fellow firefighters, it bothers you to see them trying to cope with that accident at the intersection three months ago.

Scenario A.1

Double Fatality

First Paramedic

THE INCIDENT:

The Central Township Fire Department responded to a car-tree collision in a rural part of the county. When they arrived on scene, they found that both the driver and passenger were dead. The driver was an 85-year old male and the passenger was his 82-year old wife.

The location of the accident was approximately 400 yards east of a blinking yellow/red traffic controlled intersection that frequently has accidents due to the speed on the north-south (yellow flashing light) highway. ***In fact, this same department had been dispatched to this same intersection about three months ago when a family of four had been killed.***

The engine arrived on scene first with the two firefighters. Two volunteer firefighters arrived within five minutes, shortly before the ambulance. The paramedic received permission from medical control for a dead-on-scene call for the two victims. It was necessary to use the Jaws of Life to remove both bodies, as it was a head-on crash into the tree.

It took approximately 20 minutes to extricate the two bodies, which were transported in body bags to the local hospital morgue. The total time out on scene was about one hour and thirty minutes. The victims were residents of the township and two of the firefighters thought that they knew who they were, but didn't know either very well.

YOUR ROLE IN THIS INCIDENT:

You are the paramedic from the local ambulance service. When you arrived on scene, you confirmed that both the victims obviously were dead and requested a dead-on-scene protocol. This was granted and you stayed on scene until you were directed by the medical examiner to transport the bodies to the morgue at the hospital.

In the fact phase, share any of the information provided above.

In the thought phase, share the following information: You have worked in this area for a number of years and remember hearing about it from your partner who was on the four-person fatality a few months ago at this intersection. From what you heard, you are glad that you missed that call.

In the reaction phase, share the following information: You know that the paramedics who were on that call three months ago wouldn't say any more about it than that it was a bad call. The fire chief had talked about doing a critique about that previous call and everyone was hoping that he would forget it. You don't want to say too much because you weren't on that call.

In the symptom phase share, the following information: You haven't had any symptoms because you were not on that previous call. You want to be supportive of all the firefighters and paramedics on that four-person fatality.

Scenario A.1

Double Fatality

Second Parametic

THE INCIDENT:

The Central Township Fire Department responded to a car-tree collision in a rural part of the county. When they arrived on scene, they found that both the driver and passenger were dead. The driver was an 85-year old male and the passenger was his 82-year old wife.

The location of the accident was approximately 400 yards east of a blinking yellow/red traffic controlled intersection that frequently has accidents due to the speed on the north-south (yellow flashing light) highway. ***In fact, this same department had been dispatched to this same intersection about three months ago when a family of four had been killed.***

The engine arrived on scene first with the two firefighters. Two volunteer firefighters arrived within five minutes, shortly before the ambulance. The paramedic received permission from medical control for a dead-on-scene call for the two victims. It was necessary to use the Jaws of Life to remove both bodies, as it was a head-on crash into the tree.

It took approximately 20 minutes to extricate the two bodies, which were transported in body bags to the local hospital morgue. The total time out on scene was about one hour and thirty minutes. The victims were residents of the township and two of the firefighters thought that they knew who they were, but didn't know either very well.

YOUR ROLE IN THIS INCIDENT:

Because your partner was primary medic on this call, you drove. Your only involvement was to assist in the assessment prior to the extrication and then the body removal to the hospital morgue.

In the fact phase, share any of the information provided above.

In the thought phase, share the following information: Your first thought was, "Here we go again." You thought that when you got there, the accident would be in the same place as the previous one. You were lead paramedic at the accident where the entire family was killed when their car was broad-sided by the semi-trailer.

In the reaction phase, share the following information: This accident triggered all the thoughts from the other accident. Back then, you had been able to handle the death of the parents even though their injuries were severe. It was the death of the two kids that got to you. You and your spouse have a baby about the same age as the infant and you had to take the dead infant from the firefighter to the helicopter. Immediately after you cleared the scene, you called your wife to check on the baby.

In the symptom phase, share the following information: You thought you were over that accident. You hadn't seen the infant's face in your daughter's face for two months. During this last week, however, you have been anxious when your son is taking a nap. Your wife thinks that you are over-protective and you think you probably are, too.

Firefighter Car Crash

Facilitator's Guide Sheet

THE INCIDENT:

A phone call was received from the County Sheriff's Department that two staff persons, Stan and Mary, were killed in an auto accident yesterday morning on the way to work. It was a car/deer accident on a rural two-lane highway and it appears that no one was at fault. The car was severely damaged and Stan was thrown from the car.

Stan had been in this department for over 10 years. He was a little league coach and was well liked by the other employees. He had a great sense of humor and was quite playful.

Mary was fairly new to the department. She was somewhat quiet and not as well-known but was accepted and respected by staff.

PLACE: Eastern Township Fire Department

TIME: Yesterday: 7:30 a.m.

PERSONNEL INVOLVED:	MAJOR ISSUE:	SYMPTOMS:
1. Friend who argued with Stan	Guilt	Irritable; anxious
2. Basketball and hunting friend	Shock and denial	Intrusive images
3. Female firefighter	Anger at rumors	Trouble concentrating
4. Friend of Mary	Thoughts of mortality/family	Sleep disturbance
5. Friend of Mary who turned her down for a ride	Guilt	Disturbing dreams
6. Stan's co-coach	What to tell kids?	Memory problems
7. Rookie	Feels inadequate	Sleep disturbances

POSSIBLE PROCESS QUESTIONS:

- Did the people who needed help with guilt get it? How?
- What things did the CISM team do or say to help participants make connections (e.g., did anyone offer advice or company to the rookie)?
- How did the team do with summarizing and addressing the various symptoms?
- Are regret and self-recrimination always a theme with grief? (YES)
- Did the issue of anger at the rumors come up? Was it handled well?

NOTE: *A practice debriefing for the death(s) of a colleague should be performed with care. Make sure that you have explained the event and asked participants if they have actually experienced such an event before continuing. Those individuals should be excluded from the actual role play. Even a role play of a made-up event can trigger powerful grief issues.*

Scenario A.3

Multi-Fatality House Fire

Facilitator's Guide Sheet

THE INCIDENT:

Yesterday a call came in about a house fire. By the time the first responders arrived, the house was fully involved. Neighbors were yelling that there were three small children inside.

Within minutes, all three children were found unburned but unconscious. In spite of the efforts of the firefighters and EMTs, all three children died.

It appears that the fire was caused by one of the children playing with matches.

PLACE: Western Township Fire Department

TIME: Yesterday: 7:30 p.m.

PERSONNEL INVOLVED:	THEME:	SYMPTOMS:
1. Police officer	Lost minutes of abuse; helpless	Intrusive thoughts
2. EMT #1 (5-year-old)	"I lost him;" dread of recurrence	Anxious; overprotective
3. EMT #2 (3-year-old)	Unsure of self; needs validation	Sleep disturbance
4. EMT #3 (2-year-old)	Not sure about continuing	Anger
5. Firefighter #1 (5-year-old)	Broke down; self-doubt	Flashbacks; questioning
6. Firefighter#2 (3-year-old)	Self-doubt; needs reassurance	Checking own kids
7. Firefighter #3 (2-year-old)	Doubting skills	Flashbacks
8. Firefighter #4	Worried about friends	Flashbacks to other calls
9. Firefighter #5	Crowd screaming	Overprotective

POSSIBLE PROCESS QUESTIONS:

- Did the people who needed help with guilt get it? How?
- What things did the CISM team do or say to help participants make connections?
- How did the team do with summarizing and addressing the various symptoms?
- Are regret and self-recrimination always themes with grief? (YES)
- Did the issue of anger at the rumors come up? Was it handled well?
- How did the team respond to some of the physical symptoms that the personnel brought out?

Scenario A.4

Teenager Car Crash

Facilitator's Guide Sheet

THE INCIDENT:

Last night, a Mason City police officer observed a red Toyota Celica driving erratically so he made a stop. The male driver was a 17-year-old high school senior, obviously impaired from drinking. The passenger, a high school girl who was well-known to the officer, seemed unimpaired. Not wishing to arrest the two, the officer lectured them and ordered the young woman, who owned the car, to drive her boyfriend home and then go directly home herself.

In the next hour, a severe thunderstorm swept the county. Another officer was dispatched to a reported head-on collision with multiple victims. He found the red Toyota and a full-sized sedan in the middle of the road. The occupants of the Toyota were obviously dead or seriously injured. The driver of the sedan was lying on the berm, while his female passenger was pinned under the dash. The officer informed dispatch, requested ambulances and a pumper to handle the spilled gasoline, and also called for backups from the police department.

PLACE: Mason City

TIME: Yesterday: 11:45 p.m.

PERSONNEL INVOLVED:	THEME:	SYMPTOMS:
1. Police officer (making the original stop)	Guilt	Overprotective of child
2. Rookie firefighter	Thought he was going to die	Flashbacks
3. Fire lieutenant	Guilt at relief	Overprotective
4. EMT #1	Thought he was going to die	Flashbacks
5. Veteran firefighter	Anger at being here	Irritable at daughter
6. Police sergeant	Relief	Eating everything in sight
7. EMT #2	Anger at the door	Nightmares

POSSIBLE PROCESS QUESTIONS:

- What were some of the most important themes of self-blame?
- What support came naturally from the participants
- What good things did the CISM team say to encourage support?
- Did natural supports mention a lack of intent or "I have done that, too" for the police officer?
- What teaching comments did the best job of addressing particular symptoms?

Teenager Overdose

Facilitator's Guide Sheet

THE INCIDENT:

911 received a call at approximately 4:00 p.m. of a possible cardiac arrest of a 12-year-old in a remote part of the county. The dispatcher learned that drugs might have been involved. When they arrived on scene, the fire department found an unresponsive young boy who was in cardiac arrest. Two of the firefighters began CPR and another firefighter went out to the road to direct the ambulance to the scene. The young boy was bluish in color and his eyes appeared dilated. Another boy who was with the victim said that his friend had taken some capsules they bought at school. The capsules were supposed to make you "chill out."

Although the person who sold the capsules warned against taking more than one at a time, the victim took three or four. Shortly afterward, he became unconscious and fell to the ground. While on the ground, he started foaming at the mouth and jerking his arms and legs.

The ambulance arrived on scene and assessed the patient. The paramedics were able to intubate the teenager and ventilate him. They tried to establish an IV line. Finally, the lead paramedic consulted with the ER doctor and decided to stop all efforts as the boy's body was not responding to treatment. The mother became hysterical and started blaming her son's friend for letting him take the pills. A firefighter had to restrain the mother from hitting the other young boy. Later the rescuers learned that the boy had taken methamphetamines.

PLACE: Northern Township Fire Station

TIME: Sunday: 4:00 p.m.

PERSONNEL INVOLVED:	THEME:	SYMPTOMS:
1. 911 Dispatcher	Exposed to mom's anger	Tearful; self-doubt
2. Firefighter #1 (1st on scene)	Exposed to mom's anger	Sleep disturbance
3. Firefighter #2	Angry at mom's blaming	Isolation from wife
4. Fire chief	Understanding; supportive	None
5. Firefighter #3 (traffic control)	Identification issue	Worried about brother
6. Paramedic	Too busy to think	Worried about no reaction
7. EMT	Irritated by mom, but supports team	None

POSSIBLE PROCESS QUESTIONS:

- How might the fact phase have been important in giving the "big picture"?
- Who was the most exposed to mom's anger? Who was most affected?
- What comments seemed to facilitate the mutual support within this group?
- Name some comments which seemed intuitive or empathic.
- Any issues which should be present but which did not come out?
- Name one lesson to remember from this experience.

Scenario A.6

Firefighter Suicide

Facilitator's Guide Sheet

THE INCIDENT:

A fire department with a staff of 12 on this shift was shocked to learn about the death of Joe, a firefighter for 12 years. Joe hanged himself at some point during the night.

Joe's wife left him about six weeks ago. He had been increasingly depressed and had been drinking more lately, although few people were aware of it.

The night before last, Joe went to a bar with two of the staff. They had some drinks and eventually left him there.

Yesterday morning when he didn't show up for his regular breakfast and ride to a meeting, the other firefighter thought he had just gone to the meeting early. After arriving at the meeting and discovering that Joe had not shown up, he and a co-worker were sent to Joe's house where they found the front door unlocked and Joe hanging in his bedroom. There was no suicide note.

It is now 24 hours later.

PLACE: Johnston Fire Department

TIME: Yesterday: 7:30 a.m.

PERSONNEL INVOLVED:	THEME:	SYMPTOMS:
1. Friend #1 who found the body	Conflicting sad and mad	Visual images/dreams
2. Friend #2 who found the body	Guilty	Visual images
3. Friend #3	Shaken beliefs	Lost appetite
4. Drinking buddy #1	Guilt	Intrusive thoughts
5. Drinking buddy #2	Guilt	Poor sleep; concentration
6. Jazz buddy	Sorry	Loss of interest
7. Joe's confidant	Anger/guilt	Confusion/sad
8. New member of the department	Compassion	None

POSSIBLE PROCESS QUESTIONS:

- Were the participants able to help each other deal with guilt and anger?
- Name some things the team did to address anger and guilt (e.g., was re-fragmentation necessary)?
- How did this suicide shake the beliefs of the various participants?

NOTE: *The role playing of a suicide death of a colleague may generate very intense reactions for some of the role players. Make sure that you have explained the event and asked participants if they have actually experienced such an event before starting. Those who have should be excluded from the actual role play. Even a role play of a made-up event can trigger powerful grief issues.*

Scenario A.7

Fire Chief's Son

Facilitator's Guide Sheet

THE INCIDENT:

The call was toned out to the all-volunteer fire service that also runs on medicals at 11:30 p.m. A car had missed the last S-curve six miles south of the village and hit a tree head-on. Dispatch indicated that an ambulance was en route.

The first firefighter on scene was the assistant fire chief, who immediately recognized the silver Mustang convertible belonging to the fire chief's 16-year-old son. At about the same time, he heard the fire chief announce that he was approaching the scene. The assistant chief radioed the chief and told him to return to the station and get the Jaws of Life for extrication.

As the other firefighters arrived, they were able to confirm that it was the chief's son who had been driving the car and he was dead. The assistant fire chief radioed the chief again and told him to wait at the station because the scene was under control.

The assistant fire chief then turned the scene over to another firefighter and left for the station to inform the chief and to keep him away from the scene.

PLACE: Monroe Township

TIME: Two days ago: 11:30 p.m.

PERSONNEL INVOLVED:	THEME:	SYMPTOMS:
1. Fire chief	Anger/guilt	Totally overwhelmed
2. Assistant fire chief	Anger/protectivenss	Difficulty concentrating
3. Firefighter #1	Concerned about chief	Sleep disturbance
4. Firefighter #2	Disbelief	Lack of concentration
5. Firefighter #3	Supportive of friends	Sleep/eating problems
6. Paramedic #1	Shielding the chief	None in particular
7. Paramedic #2	Supportive of firefighters	None in particular

POSSIBLE PROCESS QUESTIONS:

- The chief wants to be with his fellow firefighters for the debriefing. Should the team permit this? If not, how should the team coordinator handle this?
- What would be the decision-making process that you would follow to make the decision?
- Would the presence of the chief adversely affect the intervention?

Scenario A.8

Single Fatality Accident

Facilitator's Guide Sheet

THE INCIDENT:

A call came into the Buford Township Volunteer Fire Department about an elderly woman having chest pains and trouble breathing. Because of the size of this small community, it just so happened that one of the medically-trained fire personnel was next door when the call was received. The paramedics arrived and determined that while the woman needed to be checked out at the hospital, it was not a critical situation. They proceeded to the hospital.

After delivering the woman to the hospital, the unit started back to their regular jobs. As he neared his home, one firefighter was flagged down by a neighbor saying there was a car in the gully. Upon investigation, he found the woman's daughter unconscious and obviously dead in a crashed vehicle. The firefighter called in the scene and the Buford Fire Department was again called out.

As the units arrived, it was determined that the victim had been rushing to the hospital because of her mother's non-terminal situation. The chief was the first to arrive as backup and realized that the victim was not only the neighbor of two of his firefighters, she was the wife of a close friend. Once the Jaws of Life arrived and the body was extracted from the vehicle, two firefighters who knew the husband were released to go to his place of employment and tell him before he heard it on the news.

Buford Township is a small community in which every one knows, or is related to, everyone else. They get very few calls in general, few fatal accidents, and even fewer which are this senseless.

PLACE: Buford Township

TIME: Two days ago: 11:30 p.m.

PERSONNEL INVOLVED:

1. Fire chief
2. Assistant fire chief
3. Firefighter #1
4. Firefighter #2
5. Firefighter #3
6. Paramedic #1
7. Paramedic #2 (female)

THEME:

Concern for personnel
Grief over previous incident
How to talk with family
Overprotective
Supportive of friends
Senseless accident
Support of fire family

SYMPTOMS:

Difficulty concentrating
Distressing dreams
Sleep disturbance
Lack of concentration
None
Fear of repetition
Improved communication

POSSIBLE PROCESS QUESTIONS:

- Is there any special way to handle the special issues when almost all of the debriefees know the victim in some fashion?
- What would you do to prepare the team to handle the dynamics of this situation?
- What were some of the major grief issues expressed here?
- Did the team teach about handling grief?
- What might they have done differently?

Ambulance Crash

Facilitator's Guide Sheet

THE INCIDENT:

An ambulance from the Upston Mills Ambulance Service was dispatched to a possible cardiac arrest patient four miles south of the village limits. Because of a sudden change in the weather, the roads had become treacherous. Due to the slippery conditions, the ambulance had significantly reduced speed. Vehicles were pulling off the road and yielding right of way to the ambulance, which was using both a siren and flashing lights.

On the right-hand side of the road, a car backing out of a driveway suddenly appeared in front of the ambulance. The driver of the car didn't seem to notice that other vehicles were pulled over for the ambulance and backed out between two of them on the side of the road. The paramedic driving the ambulance attempted to avoid the accident but was unable to stop. The modular ambulance T-boned the passenger side of the car and then flipped onto its side. An 8-year-old girl sitting without a seatbelt in the front seat of the car was killed upon impact. One of the paramedics was injured in the crash. The other paramedic called for backup and triaged the scene. The older gentleman who had been driving the car appeared unhurt but disoriented.

The cardiac patient call was turned over to another ambulance service. A second ambulance, fire truck, and police car responded to the first ambulance's call for assistance.

PLACE: Upston Mills

TIME: Five days ago: 10:00 a.m.

PERSONNEL INVOLVED:	THEME:	SYMPTOMS:
1. Paramedic #1 (first ambulance)	Anger/guilt	Intrusive images of the scene
2. Paramedic #2 (first ambulance)	Blaming himself	Sleep disturbances
3. Paramedic #3	Concerned about colleagues	Vulnerability
4. Paramedic #4	Frustrated/angry	Short-tempered with people
5. Firefighter #1	Concerned about safety	Nothing in particular
6. Firefighter #2	Anger/blaming	Defensive of EMS
7. Village police officer	Anger/blaming	Nothing in particular

POSSIBLE PROCESS QUESTIONS:

- Did the first two paramedics receive support from their colleagues?
- Was the team able to effectively redirect any blaming for the event?
- Do you believe the first two paramedics should have been included in the intervention?
- If the village police officer was investigating the accident, should he/she have been involved in the intervention?
- How might this have been handled differently and why?

This scenario is designed to have the debriefing team discover several issues before the actual debriefing. It is used most effectively if someone plays the manager of the ambulance company who has invited all of the players. The team will need to evaluate who should be included and who should be dealt with separately. There are no absolute right or wrongs, merely issues to be discussed and prepared for prior to starting the debriefing.

Scenario A.10

Fire Fatalities

Facilitator's Guide Sheet

THE INCIDENT:

911 received the first call of possible fire with smoke showing in an apartment complex on the north side of town. There were numerous calls confirming the first call with some even indicating they could see flames shooting from one of the bedroom windows.

The four-firefighter engine arrived on the scene, confirmed flames showing, and indicated to incident command that two firefighters equipped with a line were going to make an entry looking for persons in the apartment.

Upon entering the apartment on the second floor, the two firefighters did a search with a thermal imaging camera, which revealed three people in the northeast bedroom. The fire was confined to that room. After gaining entry into the room, the firefighters were able to knock down the flames. Under one bed they found a small child curled up in a ball; in the closet they found two other small children huddled together. All three children were obviously dead. They continued without success to scan the apartment for other people. With the assistance of the two firefighters attacking the fire through the window from outside of the building, the scene was quickly brought under control.

PLACE: Capital City

TIME: Three days ago: 9:30 p.m.

PERSONNEL INVOLVED:	THEME:	SYMPTOMS:
1. Firefighter #1	Anger	Intrusive images
2. Firefighter #2	Anger	Sleep disturbances
3. Firefighter #3	Anger	Blaming/irritability
4. Firefighter #4	Anger	Poor sleep and lack of concentration
5. Paramedic #1	Frustrated	Nightmares
6. Paramedic #2	Anger	Hypervigilence
7. 911 Dispatcher	Compassion for victims	Grief

POSSIBLE PROCESS QUESTIONS:

- Were the firefighters who did not enter the building processing the event differently? Explain.
- Was the team able to redirect the anger during the intervention?
- Did the team address the needs of all the participants?
- Was it appropriate to have the 911 dispatcher at the intervention?
- Was the team able to suggest ways to assist the participants in dealing with their symptoms?

Scenario A.11

Firefighter Injury

Facilitator's Guide Sheet

THE INCIDENT:

Two members from the fire department dive team were assisting Engine One with a river-rescue involving a passenger trapped in a car. The car had been forced through a guardrail near the middle of the bridge by a tractor-trailer carrying steel rods. When Engine One arrived on scene, the car was hanging half on the bridge and half in the fast-moving current of the water below. As Engine One attempted to secure the vehicle in place and get the unconscious driver out of the car, there was a shift in the weight and the car plunged into the water.

Two dive team members had been dispatched on the initial call-out to the scene and arrived shortly after the car plunged into the cold water. Both divers suited up and entered the water, hoping to rescue the single passenger in the vehicle.

During the rescue effort, they succeeded in freeing the driver and one of the divers was taking him to the surface when the fast-moving current again shifted the car and pinned the other diver between a bridge piling and the car. The first diver returned underwater and discovered that the partner's oxygen tank had been crushed in the shifting of the car. The diver was trapped and appeared to be unconscious. The first diver was able to remove the partner's tank and provide oxygen as they ascended to the surface.

The second diver is in the hospital and expected to make a full recovery. The driver of the car later died. The intervention is being held on the next duty day for this crew.

PLACE: Coryville

TIME: Three days ago: 9:30 p.m.

PERSONNEL INVOLVED:

1. Firefighter #1 (diver)
2. Firefighter #2
3. Firefighter #3
4. Firefighter #4
5. Firefighter #5
6. Firefighter captain

THEME:

Guilt / self-blame
Blaming
Anger
Concern for friend
Concerned about safety
Frustrated

SYMPTOMS:

Anxiety
Agitation
Sleep problems
Nothing in particular
Flashback of a near-drowning
Loss of control

POSSIBLE PROCESS QUESTIONS:

- Was this the right time to do the intervention (the next duty day)? Should it have been earlier?
- How did the team handle it when the fifth firefighter remained silent?
- Is there support from the other firefighters for the first diver who left his partner to take the victim to the surface?

Scenario A.12

Aerial Platform Collapse

Facilitator's Guide Sheet

THE INCIDENT:

The Pleasantville Fire Department was asked to participate in the Founders' Day Celebration. The festival committee specifically asked to have the new aerial truck (properly called an aerial platform) prominently displayed in the downtown area. When the aerial platform arrived, someone from the committee suggested that it be placed in the parking lot near the three-story parking ramp.

The firefighters situated the aerial platform and extended the four outriggers. The crew was taking advantage of the opportunity as a training exercise for the department, so every effort was made to check and recheck all the procedures for setting up the rig. After it was in place, the 100-foot aerial platform was extended with no difficulty. The agenda called for the aerial platform to be raised up to the top of the parking ramp during the opening ceremony. At the appropriate time, two firefighters climbed into the platform and the operator extended the aerial device. As the operator rotated the device to approach the top floor of the parking ramp, a noise was heard from the two outriggers on the left-hand side of the vehicle. The noise grew louder until suddenly the paved area under the outriggers on that side collapsed into an underground level of the parking ramp. This caused the truck to tip and the safety device on the outrigger to collapse from the weight. The aerial platform fell into the parking lot on top of two unoccupied vehicles. One firefighter sustained a fractured tibia/fibula and the other a fractured right clavicle and forearm. The firefighter on the turntable was thrown off the rig and sustained only minor injuries.

The two local television stations were covering the opening ceremony and captured all of this on film. One of the local stations also broadcast it on a national feed.

PLACE: Pleasantville

TIME: Two weeks ago: 2:00 p.m.

PERSONNEL INVOLVED:

1. Firefighter #1
2. Firefighter #2
3. Firefighter #3
4. Firefighter #4
5. Firefighter #5
6. Fire chief

THEME:

Public embarrassment
Line of duty injury
Shock / anger
Negative media coverage
Agitation
Public embarrassment

SYMPTOMS:

Anxiety
Agitation
Sleep problems
Irrational anger
Sleep disburbance
Loss of control

POSSIBLE PROCESS QUESTIONS:

- Do you think that the long delay from the incident to the event was detrimental to the process?
- Has the news coverage affected the participants of the intervention?
- Should the fire chief be involved in the intervention?
- Do you think that the services of the team may be needed down the road regarding this event?

Scenario A.13

Firefighter Sudden Impact

Facilitator's Guide Sheet

THE INCIDENT:

Two nights ago, six medical response firefighters were sitting down to a spaghetti supper when a man kicked open the door to the common room and walked in carrying an unconscious 10-year-old boy who was bleeding profusely. He yelled "Help me! Help me!" and laid the boy on the floor. The boy was bleeding from the neck, but was so covered in blood that it was difficult to tell where he was injured.

The boy had been riding his bike a block from the station when he was hit by a car. The car was going slowly and most of the boy's injuries were minor except for a laceration to the neck which had sliced the carotid artery. No one on the scene knew any first aid. One of the neighborhood men had picked him up and run the block to the station, leaving a trail of blood all the way.

After a moment of frozen shock, followed by a moment of inefficient teamwork when several people tried to do the same things at once, the firefighters got themselves sorted out, two applying first aid and others running for equipment. Despite their best efforts, the boy had simply lost too much blood. They used their whole arsenal of techniques at the station and during transport, but the boy was pronounced dead an hour later at the ER.

The boy was a neighborhood kid they all knew. The suddenness, the unexpected location, the lack of time to orient to emergency mode, and the threatening appearance of a blood-covered, yelling man all added to the impact of this event.

PLACE: Neighborhood Fire / EMT Combined Station

TIME: Two days ago

PERSONNEL INVOLVED:	THEME:	SYMPTOMS:
1. Chief	Initially scared, confused	Jumpy, worried about self-image
2. Firefighter #1	Food-blood association	Loss of appetite, sleep
3. Firefighter #2	Identifies with child victim	Sadness, exhaustion
4. Firefighter #3	Only one not confused	Apprehension about kids
5. Firefighter #4	Very shocked, confused	Anger at self
6. Firefighter #5	Losing a kid, loss of safety	Irritable

POSSIBLE PROCESS QUESTIONS:

- What were the impact factors which made this incident critical?
- Did the participants help each other reduce second-guessing?
- Did any of them choose to keep their biggest issues private? Why?
- Were reactions affected by being post 9-11?

LAW ENFORCEMENT-BASED EXPERIENCES

Scenario B.1
Multiple Death Domestic

Scenario B.2
Suicide By Cop

Scenario B.3
Police Officer Car Crash

Scenario B.4
Police Officer Suicide

Scenario B.5
Police Chase

Scenario B.6
State Trooper Death

Scenario B.7
Officer Shot

Scenario B.8
Police Officer Murdererer

Scenario B.9
Armed Robbery Suspect Killed

Scenario B.10
Civilian Shot

Scenario B.11
Police Standoff Suicide

Scenario B.12
Accidental Shooting of an Officer By a Fellow Officer

Scenario B.1

Multiple Death Domestic

Facilitator's Guide Sheet

THE INCIDENT:

At 11:30 p.m. the 911 dispatcher received a call from what sounded like a small child who was crying. The child said that his daddy was at the house with a gun and was going to hurt mommy. The line disconnected and the dispatcher called back only to get a busy signal.

The dispatcher sent two police cars to the area. The first police officer arrived in the area and reported no light on in the house. When the second car arrived, the officer attempted to make contact. The window next to the front door was smashed. Knocking and announcing, the police officer broke into the house. The officer found a female lying on the floor near the front door. She was dressed in a nightgown and there was blood in the chest area. The officers requested additional cars, EMS, and a field supervisor. A search of the residence revealed the bodies of three children in their beds with obvious gun shot wounds to the head.

The officers heard noise from the upstairs bathroom. A man's voice indicated that he had shot his wife and children and now he was going to take his own life. The officers ordered the man to come out slowly with his hands raised. The door burst open and a male exited the bathroom firing a handgun. The officers returned fire and the man fell to the floor. EMS arrived and transported the man to the hospital, where he died in the operating room.

PLACE: Suburbia

TIME: Two days ago: 11:30 p.m.

PERSONNEL INVOLVED:	THEME:	SYMPTOMS:
1. 911 Dispatcher	Dreading the worst	Flashbacks; fear of repetition
2. Police officer #1	Identification with own family	Intrusive images; dreams
3. Police officer #2	Physical reaction to sights	Replaying images
4. Backup officer #1	Glad it was not him/her	None
5. Backup officer #2	Anger at media	None
6. Paramedic #1	Anger at perpetrator	One
7. Paramedic #2	Visual impact; identification	Confusion; isolating
8. Field supervisor	Protective towards crew	Tired; but closer to crew

POSSIBLE PROCESS QUESTIONS:

- What did this group do with the family identification issues?
- Did debriefing help strengthen any new-found unity in this group?
- What were some of the less obvious symptoms mentioned?
- What were some good facilitating comments by the CISM team?

Scenario B.1

Multiple Death Domestic

Overview

THE INCIDENT:

At 11:30 p.m. the 911 dispatcher received a call from what sounded like a small child who was crying. The child said that his daddy was at the house with a gun and was going to hurt mommy. The line disconnected and the dispatcher called back only to get a busy signal.

The dispatcher sent two police cars to the area. The first police officer arrived in the area and reported no light on in the house. When the second car arrived, the officer attempted to make contact. The window next to the front door was smashed. Knocking and announcing, the police officer broke into the house. The officer found a female lying on the floor near the front door. She was dressed in a nightgown and there was blood in the chest area. The officers requested additional cars, EMS, and a field supervisor. A search of the residence revealed the bodies of three children in their beds with obvious gun shot wounds to the head.

The officers heard noise from the upstairs bathroom. A man's voice indicated that he had shot his wife and children and now he was going to take his own life. The officers ordered the man to come out slowly with his hands raised. The door burst open and a male exited the bathroom firing a handgun. The officers returned fire and the man fell to the floor. EMS arrived and transported the man to the hospital, where he died in the operating room.

PLACE: Suburbia

TIME: Two days ago: 11:30 p.m.

PERSONNEL INVOLVED:

1. 911 Dispatcher
2. Police officer #1
3. Police officer #2
4. Backup officer #1
5. Backup officer #2
6. Paramedic #1
7. Paramedic #2
8. Field supervisor

Scenario B.1

Multiple Death Domestic

911 Dispatcher

THE INCIDENT:

At 11:30 p.m. the 911 dispatcher received a call from what sounded like a small child who was crying. The child said that his daddy was at the house with a gun and was going to hurt mommy. The line disconnected and the dispatcher called back only to get a busy signal.

The dispatcher sent two police cars to the area. The first police officer arrived in the area and reported no light on in the house. When the second car arrived, the officer attempted to make contact. The window next to the front door was smashed. Knocking and announcing, the police officer broke into the house. The officer found a female lying on the floor near the front door. She was dressed in a nightgown and there was blood in the chest area. The officers requested additional cars, EMS, and a field supervisor. A search of the residence revealed the bodies of three children in their beds with obvious gun shot wounds to the head.

The officers heard noise from the upstairs bathroom. A man's voice indicated that he had shot his wife and children and now he was going to take his own life. The officers ordered the man to come out slowly with his hands raised. The door burst open and a male exited the bathroom firing a handgun. The officers returned fire and the man fell to the floor. EMS arrived and transported the man to the hospital, where he died in the operating room.

YOUR ROLE IN THIS INCIDENT:

You received the call from the small child and dispatched the response units.

In the fact phase, share any of the information provided above.

In the thought phase, share the following information: When you got a busy signal on the call back you were afraid that something had happened to the child.

In the reaction phase, share the following information: When the officer radioed for back-up units, EMS, and a field supervisor, you knew something horrible had happened. You kept telling yourself not to imagine the worst, but that's exactly what happened.

In the symptom phase, share the following information: You had another 911 child call since this event. Even though it turned out to be a false alarm, you had to turn the call over to another 911 dispatcher because it brought the entire scene back to you. You never want to hear something like that again.

Scenario B.1

Multiple Death Domestic

First Officer on the Scene

THE INCIDENT:

At 11:30 p.m. the 911 dispatcher received a call from what sounded like a small child who was crying. The child said that his daddy was at the house with a gun and was going to hurt mommy. The line disconnected and the dispatcher called back only to get a busy signal.

The dispatcher sent two police cars to the area. The first police officer arrived in the area and reported no light on in the house. When the second car arrived, the officer attempted to make contact. The window next to the front door was smashed. Knocking and announcing, the police officer broke into the house. The officer found a female lying on the floor near the front door. She was dressed in a nightgown and there was blood in the chest area. The officers requested additional cars, EMS, and a field supervisor. A search of the residence revealed the bodies of three children in their beds with obvious gun shot wounds to the head.

The officers heard noise from the upstairs bathroom. A man's voice indicated that he had shot his wife and children and now he was going to take his own life. The officers ordered the man to come out slowly with his hands raised. The door burst open and a male exited the bathroom firing a handgun. The officers returned fire and the man fell to the floor. EMS arrived and transported the man to the hospital, where he died in the operating room.

YOUR ROLE IN THIS INCIDENT:

You arrived on scene and waited for a backup before you approached the house.

In the fact phase, share any of the information provided above.

In the thought phase, share the following information: You suspected that this was going to be a bad scene when you saw the window broken out next to the door.

In the reaction phase, share the following information: It was hard enough when you found the woman's body, but it was worse when you found the oldest boy's body. It is also difficult to be on administrative leave because you or your partner killed the man.

In the symptom phase, share the following information: When you close your eyes, you still see the face of the child that looks like your own son. You haven't slept well since that night.

Scenario B.1

Multiple Death Domestic

Second Officer on the Scene

THE INCIDENT:

At 11:30 p.m. the 911 dispatcher received a call from what sounded like a small child who was crying. The child said that his daddy was at the house with a gun and was going to hurt mommy. The line disconnected and the dispatcher called back only to get a busy signal.

The dispatcher sent two police cars to the area. The first police officer arrived in the area and reported no light on in the house. When the second car arrived, the officer attempted to make contact. The window next to the front door was smashed. Knocking and announcing, the police officer broke into the house. The officer found a female lying on the floor near the front door. She was dressed in a nightgown and there was blood in the chest area. The officers requested additional cars, EMS, and a field supervisor. A search of the residence revealed the bodies of three children in their beds with obvious gun shot wounds to the head.

The officers heard noise from the upstairs bathroom. A man's voice indicated that he had shot his wife and children and now he was going to take his own life. The officers ordered the man to come out slowly with his hands raised. The door burst open and a male exited the bathroom firing a handgun. The officers returned fire and the man fell to the floor. EMS arrived and transported the man to the hospital, where he died in the operating room.

YOUR ROLE IN THIS INCIDENT:

You and the first officer gained entry to the house and found the woman's body. You also found the bodies of two of the children in their bedrooms.

In the fact phase, share any of the information provided above.

In the thought phase, share the following information: You keep wishing that the man had killed himself instead of his wife and children. Why did they have to suffer for his problems?

In the reaction phase, share the following information: The worst part was definitely the sight of the two small children. At first, you thought they were asleep until you noticed the gunshot wounds to their heads. You came close to vomiting, but you knew that you had to find the shooter of these small children.

In the symptom phase, share the following information: You have no regrets for having shot the man, yet you still have flashbacks of him shooting at you.

Multiple Death Domestic

First Backup Officer

THE INCIDENT:

At 11:30 p.m. the 911 dispatcher received a call from what sounded like a small child who was crying. The child said that his daddy was at the house with a gun and was going to hurt mommy. The line disconnected and the dispatcher called back only to get a busy signal.

The dispatcher sent two police cars to the area. The first police officer arrived in the area and reported no light on in the house. When the second car arrived, the officer attempted to make contact. The window next to the front door was smashed. Knocking and announcing, the police officer broke into the house. The officer found a female lying on the floor near the front door. She was dressed in a nightgown and there was blood in the chest area. The officers requested additional cars, EMS, and a field supervisor. A search of the residence revealed the bodies of three children in their beds with obvious gun shot wounds to the head.

The officers heard noise from the upstairs bathroom. A man's voice indicated that he had shot his wife and children and now he was going to take his own life. The officers ordered the man to come out slowly with his hands raised. The door burst open and a male exited the bathroom firing a handgun. The officers returned fire and the man fell to the floor. EMS arrived and transported the man to the hospital, where he died in the operating room.

YOUR ROLE IN THIS INCIDENT:

You arrived and set up the crime scene. You never entered the house.

In the fact phase, share any of the information provided above.

In the thought phase, share the following information: Your first thoughts were imagining the scene described by the first officer on scene. You still can't understand why he and his partner are on administrative leave for killing the man.

In the reaction phase, share the following information: You know that the scene has been difficult for the first two officers on scene. You keep thinking that if you hadn't made a traffic stop a few minutes before this event that you would have been the first officer on scene because you were closer to the scene. Secretly, you're not sure *how* you feel about that.

In the symptom phase, share the following information: You haven't noticed any disruptions in your normal routine.

Scenario B.1

Multiple Death Domestic

Second Backup Officer

THE INCIDENT:

At 11:30 p.m. the 911 dispatcher received a call from what sounded like a small child who was crying. The child said that his daddy was at the house with a gun and was going to hurt mommy. The line disconnected and the dispatcher called back only to get a busy signal.

The dispatcher sent two police cars to the area. The first police officer arrived in the area and reported no light on in the house. When the second car arrived, the officer attempted to make contact. The window next to the front door was smashed. Knocking and announcing, the police officer broke into the house. The officer found a female lying on the floor near the front door. She was dressed in a nightgown and there was blood in the chest area. The officers requested additional cars, EMS, and a field supervisor. A search of the residence revealed the bodies of three children in their beds with obvious gun shot wounds to the head.

The officers heard noise from the upstairs bathroom. A man's voice indicated that he had shot his wife and children and now he was going to take his own life. The officers ordered the man to come out slowly with his hands raised. The door burst open and a male exited the bathroom firing a handgun. The officers returned fire and the man fell to the floor. EMS arrived and transported the man to the hospital, where he died in the operating room.

YOUR ROLE IN THIS INCIDENT:

Along with the first backup officer, your responsibility was to secure the crime scene. This job was made more difficult because somehow the media found out about the event and came on scene with their cameras.

In the fact phase, share any of the information provided above.

In the thought phase, share the following information: You have always had a difficult time with the intrusion of the media at crime scenes.

In the reaction phase, share the following information: The news reporters wanted to interview the two officers who were involved with the shooting. You could imagine how your co-workers might feel and you were really angry at those reporters. You will always remember with pleasure how the field supervisor dealt with those jerks.

In the symptom phase, share the following information: You haven't observed any unusual symptoms, except that you can't watch the local news without making insulting comments to the reporters on screen. Your spouse is tired of hearing it, so you just don't watch the news anymore.

Scenario B.1

Multiple Death Domestic

First Paramedic

THE INCIDENT:

At 11:30 p.m. the 911 dispatcher received a call from what sounded like a small child who was crying. The child said that his daddy was at the house with a gun and was going to hurt mommy. The line disconnected and the dispatcher called back only to get a busy signal.

The dispatcher sent two police cars to the area. The first police officer arrived in the area and reported no light on in the house. When the second car arrived, the officer attempted to make contact. The window next to the front door was smashed. Knocking and announcing, the police officer broke into the house. The officer found a female lying on the floor near the front door. She was dressed in a nightgown and there was blood in the chest area. The officers requested additional cars, EMS, and a field supervisor. A search of the residence revealed the bodies of three children in their beds with obvious gun shot wounds to the head.

The officers heard noise from the upstairs bathroom. A man's voice indicated that he had shot his wife and children and now he was going to take his own life. The officers ordered the man to come out slowly with his hands raised. The door burst open and a male exited the bathroom firing a handgun. The officers returned fire and the man fell to the floor. EMS arrived and transported the man to the hospital, where he died in the operating room.

YOUR ROLE IN THIS INCIDENT:

You treated the man who had been shot by the police.

In the fact phase, share any of the information provided above.

In the thought phase, share the following information: You were thankful that both police officers were wearing their Kevlar vests. Your patient was in bad shape with at least three shots to the chest area.

In the reaction phase, share the following information: You are angry that your patient, who was apparently responsible for the death of his wife and children, must be treated with professional respect. This may have been a bad scene visually, but from the standpoint of stressful decisions, this one did not have any for you.

In the symptom phase, share the following information: You haven't noticed any unusual symptoms.

You may be in a position to offer positive support to others.

Scenario B.1

Multiple Death Domestic

Second Paramedic

THE INCIDENT:

At 11:30 p.m. the 911 dispatcher received a call from what sounded like a small child who was crying. The child said that his daddy was at the house with a gun and was going to hurt mommy. The line disconnected and the dispatcher called back only to get a busy signal.

The dispatcher sent two police cars to the area. The first police officer arrived in the area and reported no light on in the house. When the second car arrived, the officer attempted to make contact. The window next to the front door was smashed. Knocking and announcing, the police officer broke into the house. The officer found a female lying on the floor near the front door. She was dressed in a nightgown and there was blood in the chest area. The officers requested additional cars, EMS, and a field supervisor. A search of the residence revealed the bodies of three children in their beds with obvious gun shot wounds to the head.

The officers heard noise from the upstairs bathroom. A man's voice indicated that he had shot his wife and children and now he was going to take his own life. The officers ordered the man to come out slowly with his hands raised. The door burst open and a male exited the bathroom firing a handgun. The officers returned fire and the man fell to the floor. EMS arrived and transported the man to the hospital, where he died in the operating room.

YOUR ROLE IN THIS INCIDENT:

You checked the bodies of the woman downstairs and the three children while your partner worked on the man the police shot.

In the fact phase, share any of the information provided above.

In the thought phase, share the following information: You keep thinking of how at one time this was a loving and caring family. You wonder what went so wrong.

In the reaction phase, share the following information: Although you have seen many bad scenes, this one is the worst you have ever worked. You noticed that it appeared to you that the older boy was trying to protect himself. The other two appeared to have been shot in their sleep. You and your wife are expecting your first child and you are wondering how a loving relationship could end this way.

In the symptom phase, share the following information: You keep seeing the faces of the small children whenever you try to sleep. You haven't been yourself lately and you know that you have been difficult towards your wife. You just need to sort things out.

Scenario B.1

Multiple Death Domestic

Field Supervisor

THE INCIDENT:

At 11:30 p.m. the 911 dispatcher received a call from what sounded like a small child who was crying. The child said that his daddy was at the house with a gun and was going to hurt mommy. The line disconnected and the dispatcher called back only to get a busy signal.

The dispatcher sent two police cars to the area. The first police officer arrived in the area and reported no light on in the house. When the second car arrived, the officer attempted to make contact. The window next to the front door was smashed. Knocking and announcing, the police officer broke into the house. The officer found a female lying on the floor near the front door. She was dressed in a nightgown and there was blood in the chest area. The officers requested additional cars, EMS, and a field supervisor. A search of the residence revealed the bodies of three children in their beds with obvious gun shot wounds to the head.

The officers heard noise from the upstairs bathroom. A man's voice indicated that he had shot his wife and children and now he was going to take his own life. The officers ordered the man to come out slowly with his hands raised. The door burst open and a male exited the bathroom firing a handgun. The officers returned fire and the man fell to the floor. EMS arrived and transported the man to the hospital, where he died in the operating room.

YOUR ROLE IN THIS INCIDENT:

You arrived on scene just after the shooting, at the same time as the paramedics, and just before the reporters. You hadn't even had time to hear the story from your own officers yet and were still very worried about your personnel when you had to interrupt everything to deal with those reporters, who acted if they were going to take their cameras right into the house! You almost lost it. You put on your "drill sergeant" voice and placed them behind the new perimeter—over a block away. You wouldn't give them any information at all.

In the fact phase, share any of the information provided above.

In the thought phase, share the following information: Your first thought was, "If I find out that one of my officers has been lying injured while I've had to deal with reporters, I am going to either shoot or arrest them!"

In the reaction phase, share the following information: You are feeling very protective of your officers. You are angry that young officers had to be exposed to such a bad scene. You are proud at how they handled themselves. You are very angry with the media. You feel much closer to some of the personnel who were on site.

In the symptom phase, share the following information: You have some continuing anger over the whole media issue. You often feel defensive when answering even routine questions for the department. In general, you just feel tired all the time.

Scenario B.2

Suicide By Cop

Facilitator's Guide Sheet

THE INCIDENT:

911 received a call of shots fired. Two patrol units and the command officer were dispatched to the scene. The first officer arrived and saw a woman frantically waving her hands. Just as the officer got out of the car, he heard a shot fired and felt a burning sensation in his left upper shoulder, knocking him to the ground. He radioed "officer down" and crawled behind his patrol car. He was able to determine that the shot came from the second floor window of a nearby house.

The command officer arrived and was able to get safely to the injured officer and determine that the wound didn't appear life threatening. The command officer telephoned the house and a woman told him that she had tried to wave the police officer away because her 17-year-old son was in the second floor window with a rifle. She explained that he had shot his father and threatened to kill himself. When questioned further, she stated that the son appeared high on drugs when he came home and became angry when they told him to leave the house or they would call the police.

As the command officer talked with the mother, he noticed the young man appear at the window pointing a rifle towards the officers below. Using the police car P.A. system, the command officer ordered him to drop the gun. When the young man fired, the command officer returned fire. The young man dropped the gun and fell backwards into the room.

On orders of the command officer, the perimeter officers rushed the house. They found the body of the young man in the second floor bedroom. There were no more live rounds in the rifle. The father was still alive, although seriously injured. Police officers also found a suicide note on the young man's computer stating that he had been trying to get up enough nerve to kill himself since he found out that he was HIV positive.

PLACE: North Side Precinct

TIME: Saturday morning: 2:30 a.m.

PERSONNEL INVOLVED:	THEME:	SYMPTOMS:
1. 911 Dispatcher	Anxiety about information	Jumpy
2. Command officer	Second-guessing decisions	Intrusive images
3. Police officer #1	Thinking about mortality	Intrusive images
4. Police officer #2	Wife is anxious	Increased drinking
5. Police officer #3	Second-guessing self	Irritable; isolating self
6. Police officer #4	Never had a clue	Will be more cautious

POSSIBLE PROCESS QUESTIONS:

- How did the CISM team get the participants to confront the second-guessing?
- What did this group do with the family concerns issue?
- What were some "silver lining" or adaptive outcomes of this event?
- Who may have gotten the most relief or reassurance from this debriefing?
- What good "teaching around symptoms" did you notice?

Scenario B.3

Police Officer Car Crash

Facilitator's Guide Sheet

THE INCIDENT:

A phone call was received from the county sheriff's department that two officers, Stan and Mary, were killed in an auto accident yesterday morning on the way to work. It was a car/deer accident on a rural two-lane highway and it appears that no one was at fault.

The car was severely damaged and Stan was thrown from the car. Stan had been in this department for over 10 years. He was one of the coaches for a little league team team and was well liked by all. He had a great sense of humor and was quite playful.

Mary was fairly new to the department. She was somewhat quiet and not as well-known, but was accepted and respected by the staff.

The following officers are brought together because of their close association with the victims.

PLACE: Bragg Township Police Department

TIME: Yesterday: 7:30 a.m.

PERSONNEL INVOLVED:	THEME:	SYMPTOMS:
1. Friend who argued with Stan	Guilt	Irritable; anxious
2. Stan's basketball and hunting friend	Shock and denial	Intrusive images
3. Female police officer	Anger at rumors	Trouble concentrating
4. Friend of Mary	Thoughts of mortality and family	Sleep disturbance
5. Friend who turned down Mary for a ride	Guilt	Disturbing dreams
6. Stan's co-coach and fellow officer	What to tell the kids?	Memory problems
7. Rookie officer	Feels inadequate	Sleep disturbances

POSSIBLE PROCESS QUESTIONS:

- Did the people who needed help with guilt get it? How?
- What things did the CISM team do or say to help participants make connections (e.g., did anyone offer advice or company to the rookie)?
- How did the team do with summarizing and addressing the various symptoms?
- Is regret and self-recrimination always a theme with grief? (YES)
- Did the issues around anger get handled? How?

NOTE: *A practice debriefing for the death(s) of a colleague should be performed with care. Make sure that you have explained the event and asked participants if they have actually experienced such an event before continuing. Those individuals should be excluded from the actual role play. Even a role play of a made-up event can trigger powerful grief issues.*

Scenario B.4

Police Officer Suicide

Facilitator's Guide Sheet

THE INCIDENT:

A police department with a staff of 12 on this shift was shocked to learn about the death of Joe, a police officer for 12 years. Joe hanged himself at some point during the night.

Joe's wife had left him about six weeks ago. He had been increasingly depressed and had been drinking more lately, although few people were aware of it.

The night before last, Joe went to a bar with two staff members. They had some drinks and eventually left him there.

Yesterday morning when he didn't show up for his regular breakfast and ride to a meeting, the other police officer thought he had just gone to the meeting early. After arriving at the meeting and discovering that Joe had not shown up, he and a co-worker went to Joe's house where they found the front door unlocked and Joe hanging in his bedroom. There was no suicide note.

It is now 24 hours later.

PLACE: Johnston Police Department

TIME: Yesterday: 7:30 a.m.

PERSONNEL INVOLVED:	THEME:	SYMPTOMS:
1. Friend # 1 who found body	Guilty	Visual images
4. Friend #2 who found body	Conflicting sad and mad	Visual images/dreams
2. Friend #3	Shaken beliefs	Lost appetite
3. Drinking buddy	Guilt	Intrusive thoughts
5. Jazz buddy	Sorry	Loss of interest
6. Joe's confidant	Anger/guilt	Confusion/sad
7. Rookie officer	Compassion	None
8. Drinking buddy	Guilt	Poor sleep; concentration

POSSIBLE PROCESS QUESTIONS:

- Were the participants able to help each other deal with guilt and anger?
- Name some things the team did to address anger and guilt (e.g., was re-fragmentation necessary)?
- How did this suicide shake the beliefs of the various participants?

***NOTE:** The role playing of a suicide death of a colleague may generate very intense reactions for some of the role players. Make sure that you have explained the event and asked participants if they have actually experienced such an event. Those who have should be excluded from the actual role play. Even a role play of a made-up event can trigger powerful grief issues.*

Scenario B.5

Police Chase

Facilitator's Guide Sheet

THE INCIDENT:

While a police officer was writing a ticket to a speeding motorist on the outskirts of town, she observed a car driving in an erratic fashion. Just as she finished with the speeder, she observed the car again. She decided to make a stop and check out the driver. Her patrol car was facing the opposite direction and so she turned on the overhead lights and made a U-turn.

The driver of the car observed the lights come on and increased speed to elude the officer. The chase lasted for less than two city blocks when the driver turned onto the exit ramp of the expressway. The officer followed, turning on the siren to warn the oncoming traffic.

The eluding car entered the expressway and collided with a semi-trailer head-on, killing the driver of the car instantly. The driver was a 17-year-old who had been suspended from school that morning, had been drinking, and had stolen the car. It appeared as though he panicked when the officer attempted to stop him.

Three days have passed and the accident investigation by the county sheriff's department is complete.

PLACE: Beckwith City

TIME: Three days ago: 10:00 a.m.

PERSONNEL INVOLVED:	THEME:	SYMPTOMS:
1. Police officer #1 (female)	Anger/guilt	Intrusive thoughts
2. Police officer #2	Anger/defensive	None in particular
3. Police officer #3	Concerned about friend	Intrusive image
4. Firefighter #1	Frustrated	Poor sleep; concentration
5. Firefighter #2	Supportive of friends	Overprotective of son
6. Paramedic	Concerned for police officer	None in particular
7. EMT	Compassion for victim	Reliving the scene at night in bed

POSSIBLE PROCESS QUESTIONS:

- Were the other officers' and EMS personnel's comments beneficial in helping the police officer deal with her guilt and anger?
- Was the team able to expand on the participants' support for the police officer during the teaching and re-entry phases?
- Did the team address the needs of all the participants?

Scenario B.6

State Trooper Death

Facilitator's Guide Sheet

THE INCIDENT:

A state trooper was dispatched to an area on the interstate that runs near the city center. Upon arrival, he found a stalled vehicle in the right lane. He placed his patrol car behind the stalled car and activated the flashing lights.

He approached the vehicle on the driver side. A car attempted to change lanes to pass the parked patrol car, but traffic in the left lane wouldn't let the car in. The driver tried to avoid an accident and swerved back into the right lane, hitting the state trooper and dragging his body several yards down the interstate. The trooper's body dislodged from the car and was lying in the right lane. The car, however, did not stop.

The owner of the stalled motor vehicle was able to obtain the other car's license plate number. When the sheriff's deputy went to the residence of the suspect, he found the car parked in the driveway with damage to the right fender and front door. The owner of the car indicated that she was driving on the interstate in that area, remembered the patrol car parked with its lights flashing, but didn't know that she had hit anything.

PLACE: Interstate Highway

TIME: Four days ago: 5:30 p.m.

PERSONNEL INVOLVED:	THEME:	SYMPTOMS:
1. City officer #1	Anger	Vulnerability
2. City officer #2	Anger	Disbelief
3. County deputy #1	Loss of a fellow officer	Intrusive images
4. County deputy #2	Anger	Lack of concentration
5. Firefighter #1	Safety of scene	None in particular
6. Firefighter #2	Safety of rescuers	None in particular
7. Paramedic #1	Concern for privacy	None in particular
8. Paramedic #2	Frustration in waiting	Sleep disturbance

POSSIBLE PROCESS QUESTIONS:

- What techniques could a team use to deal with the anger issue?
- How can a team keep the debriefing focused when there are several major issues?
- How can a team assure the participants that what is said in the room should stay in the room? Give some examples.

Scenario B.7

Officer Shot

Facilitator's Guide Sheet

THE INCIDENT:

A local police officer from Cedar Valley was delivering a PPO (Personal Protection Order) to an ex-live-in boyfriend. The woman had obtained the order because her former boyfriend was continuing to harass and threaten her at work and where she was staying.

The police officer approached the home of the ex-boyfriend and was surprised to see him opening the door with a gun in his hand. The police officer drew his service revolver and started moving backward to his car to radio for a backup unit. The officer almost made it to the vehicle when he heard a shot and felt a burning sensation in his upper chest. The police officer radioed an "officer down" message and stayed behind the door of the vehicle. The ex-boyfriend approached the vehicle still pointing his gun and the police officer ordered him to drop the gun. When the man refused, the officer shot and killed him.

Three other city police cars, one detective's car, and a deputy sheriff arrived on scene to assist their fellow officer who by then was unconscious. The paramedics arrived and transported him to the hospital where he underwent surgery and had a bullet removed from his chest. He is still in guarded condition.

PLACE: Cedar Valley

TIME: Two days ago: 9:30 a.m.

PERSONNEL INVOLVED:

1. Police officer #1
2. Police officer #2
3. Police officer #3
4. Police detective
5. Sheriff's deputy
6. 911 Dispatcher #1
7. 911 Dispatcher #2

THEME:

Disbelief
Frustration
Guilt
Confusion
Vulnerability
Helplessness
Fear for officer safety

SYMPTOMS:

Hyper-vigilance
Blaming
Apprehension
Hyper-alert
Concern for victim
Fear and worry
Sleep disturbances

POSSIBLE PROCESS QUESTIONS:

- How did the team handle previous issues that came up during this intervention?
- Was there any problem with the mix of police officers, deputy sheriff, and 911 dispatchers?
- Did the team address the needs of all the participants?
- Would you suspect that follow-up would be needed with any of the participants?

Scenario B.8

Police Officer Murderer

Facilitator's Guide Sheet

THE INCIDENT:

911 received a call of shots fired in the Foley Public Relations Office on Division Street. Four officers and a sergeant were dispatched to the scene. The first officer arrived and saw a woman frantically waving her hands. She indicated that a police officer was in the office and had just shot his estranged wife. The second officer arrived and the two officers cautiously began to enter the offices. As they came around a corner, they saw a woman lying in a pool of blood and a uniformed officer, Bob Smith, standing at the far end of the hallway with a drawn weapon in his hand. They yelled at him to drop his weapon, at which time he brought it up and fired. He then ducked into an office and barricaded the door.

The command officer arrived and made sure all exits were covered. He then established contact with the barricaded officer and was able to get him to surrender. The officer was taken into custody and booked into jail.

The entire department was shocked to hear what happened, especially since the officer was a 12-year veteran and considered by all to be a good cop. This was his second wife and no one was aware that a divorce was imminent.

It is now 30 hours later.

PLACE: South Side Precinct

TIME: Tuesday: Noon

PERSONNEL INVOLVED:

1. 911 Dispatcher
2. Command officer
3. Police officer #1
4. Police officer #2
5. Police officer #3
6. Police officer #4

THEME:

Anxiety about information
Second-guessing decisions
Thinking about mortality
Wife is anxious
Second guessing self
Angry at public and at Bob

SYMPTOMS:

Jumpy; anxious
Numbness; shock
Intrusive images
Increased drinking
Irritable; isolating self
Will be more cautious

POSSIBLE PROCESS QUESTIONS:

- How was the issue of guilt handled by the group? By the CISM team?
- How did the CISM team get the participants to confront the second-guessing?
- What were some "silver lining" or adaptive outcomes of this event?
- How did the CISM team facilitate these?
- Who may have gotten the most relief or reassurance from this debriefing?
- What good teaching did the team provide, especially about symptoms?

Scenario B.9

Armed Robbery Suspect Killed

Facilitator's Guide Sheet

THE INCIDENT:

The police were called to an all-night convenience store on the east side of town which had had three armed robberies in the last month. The dispatcher indicated that the suspects were seen traveling southbound on 14th Street in a white car.

As units approached the corner of 14th Street and Main, they observed a white car being driven in an erratic manner turning onto Main Street. The first officer turned on the overheads and siren and attempted to stop the vehicle. The vehicle sped off. The officer called for backup units.

After a short pursuit, the suspect vehicle pulled off the road and the driver and two passengers bailed out of the car. The first officer pursued the driver. Another officer and the sheriff's deputy chased the two other suspects. The fleeing driver turned around and pointed something at the police officer. The police officer thought it was a gun, shouted the normal police warning, and got a shot off, which killed the suspect. The suspect appeared to be approximately 14 years of age. It was discovered that the suspect's gun was a look-alike toy gun.

PLACE: Cloverdale

TIME: Three days ago: 2:30 a.m.

PERSONNEL INVOLVED:	THEME:	SYMPTOMS:
1. Police officer #1	Guilt	Physical tremors
2. Police officer #2	Defensive	None in particular
3. Police officer #3	Protect the blue line	Intrusive image
4. Police chief	Need for investigation	Concerned about public opinion
5. Sheriff's deputy	Interagency backup	Anxious and irritable

POSSIBLE PROCESS QUESTIONS:

- Was the officer who shot the 14-year-old being supported by his fellow officers?
- Should the police chief have been involved in the intervention, considering he was not on scene?
- Did the inclusion of the chief have any positive or negative effect on the officers?

Scenario B.10

Civilian Shot

Facilitator's Guide Sheet

THE INCIDENT:

Four nights ago, during a very foggy third watch, dispatch received an urgent radio call from a security guard at a storage warehouse saying that he had interrupted a break-in and had been shot. His wound wasn't critical and he was able to relay a description of the perpetrator as a white male in his 20's with a ponytail, driving a late model black Jeep with no license plates. A broadcast went out immediately.

Ten minutes later, a lone officer in a patrol car spotted a Jeep that matched the description and began to follow it. Although it was very hard to make out details in the fog, he could not see a license plate and called in that he was making a stop, asking for backup. The Jeep pulled over and almost immediately a white male with long hair emerged, holding up an arm to shield his eyes from the officer's headlights. The officer followed procedures, but despite repeated commands to show his hands, etc., the suspect reached back into his car, emerged with an object in his hand, and began to approach the officer. After several shouted warnings and fearing for his own safety, the officer finally fired one shot and dropped the suspect who had never said one word.

Later it was revealed that this was a local college student, driving a dark green Jeep with only dealer plates in the window, on his way home a little drunk from a party. He would eventually recover from his wound and later stated that he had reached into his car to get his wallet. He had approached the police cruiser so fast "to show that I was cooperating" and hadn't answered any commands because "I was afraid I'd sound drunk." Later investigation corroborated the officer's version of events and found the shooting to be justified.

PLACE: A Small City Police Department

TIME: Four days ago

PERSONNEL INVOLVED:	THEME:	SYMPTOMS:
1. Police officer #1	Sense of responsibility	Distracted, preoccupied
2. Police officer #2	Secret relief, creeped out	Jumpy and over-viligant
3. Police officer #3	Concern for fellow officer	None
4. Sergeant supervisor	Responsibility, role conflict	Feeling isolated
5. Lt. watch commander	Role conflict	Feeling isolated
6. Dispatcher	Unable to help	Over-protective, worried

POSSIBLE PROCESS QUESTIONS:

- Did this group have trouble avoiding critiquing? How did the team limit that?
- Discuss the pro's and con's of having the command staff and the shooting officer in the group. Were the sergeant and lieutenant able to discuss their personal reactions?
- Name some things said in the group which may lead to better department morale.
- Did the discussion help the officers plan how to support their fellow officer who shot the innocent victim?

Scenario B.11

Police Standoff Suicide

Facilitator's Guide Sheet

THE INCIDENT:

Yesterday evening, the 911 operator received a call that a man had gone berserk, slashed several family members with a butcher knife, and was now barricaded inside his house. The first officers to arrive observed the man moving throughout the house, yelling bizarre things about the devil, and throwing furniture through the windows. They called in and the SWAT unit was deployed.

Over the next two hours, very little communication was established and that was only through yelling. The suspect claimed to have a gun, but never fired one. Family members said it was possible, but they had not seen it. There was discussion and some disagreement about whether or not to take the suspect forcefully.

Suddenly an upstairs bedroom erupted in flames. The suspect was seen running from window to window in the affected room, yelling and laughing, waving the butcher knife, and screaming that the police were devils who wouldn't get him. When his clothes caught fire, he jumped through the window and fell to the pavement, mercifully knocking himself unconscious. He died of his injuries a short time later in the ER. It was later learned that he had doused himself with the same accelerant he had used to start the fire and that he had burns over 90% of his body.

PLACE: A Small City Police Department

TIME: One day ago

PERSONNEL INVOLVED:	THEME:	SYMPTOMS:
1. Police officer #1	Horror at own thoughts	Intrusive images, smell
2. Police officer #2	Confusion at unreality	No sleep, smell imprint
3. SWAT officer #1	Anger at suspect	Images and smells
4. SWAT officer #2	Frustrated and angry	Irritable
5. SWAT officer #3	Angry, protective of unit	No symptoms
6. SWAT sergeant	Stressed by screams	No sleep, appetite
7. Lieutenant	Concern for men, public image	Disturbing images
8. EMT #1	Touching the body	Feels contaminated
9. EMT #2	Disturbed by insanity	No symptoms, supportive

POSSIBLE PROCESS QUESTIONS:

- Was 24 hours "okay" timing for this one?
- Were there any problems with mixing units, departments, and ranks?
- This one had lots of sensory imprinting. Did the team do some good education on flashbacks?
- How did the team encourage mutual support, advice-giving, etc.?
- Do you think this discussion would have been unifying for the police department as a whole?
- Did the group help each other come to grips with the disturbing nature of the suspect's behavior?

Scenario B.12

Accidental Shooting of an Officer by a Fellow Officer

Facilitator's Guide Sheet

THE INCIDENT:

At 12:15 a.m., 911 dispatch received a cell phone call of an armed robbery in progress from a customer in a car in front of a convenience store. The dispatcher sent one primary car, two backup cars, and the zone commander. The primary car arrived in front of the store and directed the two backup cars to establish a perimeter, covering the back door and the other exit from the parking area. The primary officer, using the public address system on his car, ordered the gunmen to lay down their arms and exit the front of the store one person at a time. The lights in the store were extinguished and came back on. At that point, a gunshot was heard from within the store.

A rookie officer who was covering the back door saw movement of the door and ordered the person to throw out his/her firearm. A woman opened the door and held up her arms. She told the officer she was the owner's wife and that she was letting the police in through the back door. The rookie entered the back door and was guided through the storeroom to the door to the main store. The woman told the officer that there were two men with guns and that three customers were in the store at the time of the robbery. They had been ordered to the floor by the robbers.

The woman was able to turn on the lights in the main store from the storeroom and the rookie entered the main store area. He saw the two gunmen near the cash register. He pointed his gun in their direction and ordered them to throw down their guns. One of the robbers ran for the front door. As he exited, the other robber fired a shot at the rookie officer who ducked behind a shelf unit. The primary officer, believing that the exiting robber was firing at him, returned fire. The bullet entered the store and the ricochet hit the rookie officer in the shoulder.

The other police unit and zone commander arrived, secured the scene, and took the two men into custody. An ambulance transported the injured rookie police officer. The rookie was treated and released from the hospital with a minor gunshot injury.

PLACE: Meadstown

TIME: Six days ago: 12:15 a.m.

PERSONNEL INVOLVED:

1. Police officer #1
2. Rookie police officer #2
3. Police officer #3
4. Zone commander

THEME:

Self-blaming / guilt
Inexperience
Disbelief
Frustration

SYMPTOMS:

Withdrawal
Fear / embarrassment
Hyperalert to environment
Irritability

POSSIBLE PROCESS QUESTIONS:

- Should the rookie officer be in the debriefing?
- What would you need to know to make this decision?
- How did the participants deal with the issues with the rookie officer present?
- Did this incident alter the dynamics of the participants to one another?
- How many debriefers should be helping in this event?
- How do you space yourselves in the circle if there are more than two of you?

SCHOOL-BASED EXPERIENCES

Scenario C.1

Father Seeking Child

Facilitator's Guide Sheet

THE INCIDENT:

Yesterday morning at 10:00 a.m., the non-custodial father of a fifth grader came into the school demanding that his son be released to him. When the principal refused to release the child or to identify his location, the father pulled out a gun and forced the principal to walk through the building to his son's classroom.

The principal stalled for time, knowing that the police had been called. When the police arrived, the father ran out of the building and began shooting back at the police. In the ensuing gun battle, the father was killed.

PLACE: Forest Middle School

TIME: Yesterday: 10:00 a.m.

PERSONNEL INVOLVED:	THEME:	SYMPTOMS:
1. Principal	Thoughts of mortality	Much closer to family
2. Vice principal	Self-doubts; wants reassurance	Poor concentration
3. Secretary	Helpless; slow-motion perception	Husband wants her to quit
4. Teacher #1	Second-guessing self	Intrusive flashbacks
5. Teacher #2	Fears others may blame	Flashback to Vietnam
6. Teacher #3	Anger over loss of safety	Nightmares; flashbacks
7. Teacher #4	Anger over loss of safety	Anxious; over-protective
8. School social worker	Worries about adequacy	Trying to get prepared
9. P.E. teacher	Mortality; worried about blame	Sleep disturbance

POSSIBLE PROCESS QUESTIONS:

- Who were the people needing reassurance? Did they get it? How?
- How did the issue of loss of personal safety get expressed and dealt with?
- Summarize a few good pieces of advice or teaching about managing flashbacks and nightmares.
- What were some of the good coping responses shared by the participants?
- What comments or questions could the CISM team make to facilitate more discussion of positive coping outcomes?

Father Seeking Child

Overview

THE INCIDENT:

Yesterday morning at 10:00 a.m., the non-custodial father of a fifth grader came into the school demanding that his son be released to him. When the principal refused to release the child or to identify his location, the father pulled out a gun and forced the principal to walk through the building to his son's classroom.

The principal stalled for time, knowing that the police had been called. When the police arrived, the father ran out of the building and began shooting back at the police. In the ensuing gun battle, the father was killed.

PLACE: Forest Middle School

TIME: Yesterday: 10:00 a.m.

PERSONNEL INVOLVED:

1. Principal
2. Vice principal
3. Secretary
4. Teacher #1
5. Teacher #2
6. Teacher #3
7. Teacher #4
8. School social worker
9. P.E. teacher

POSSIBLE PROCESS QUESTIONS:

- Who were the people needing reassurance? Did they get it? How?
- How did the issue of loss of personal safety get expressed and dealt with?
- Summarize a few good pieces of advice or teaching about managing flashbacks and nightmares.
- What were some of the good coping responses shared by the participants?
- What comments or questions could the CISM team make to facilitate more discussion of positive coping outcomes?

Scenario C.1

Father Seeking Child

Principal

THE INCIDENT:

Yesterday morning at 10:00 a.m., the non-custodial father of a fifth grader came into the school demanding that his son be released to him. When the principal refused to release the child or to identify his location, the father pulled out a gun and forced the principal to walk through the building to his son's classroom.

The principal stalled for time, knowing that the police had been called. When the police arrived, the father ran out of the building and began shooting back at the police. In the ensuing gun battle, the father was killed.

YOUR ROLE IN THIS INCIDENT:

You were immediately involved in the incident from start to finish. You were on "auto pilot" throughout the incident and afterward. You organized the incident response team to respond yesterday and saw to their operations today. You have been running on adrenaline and are now realizing how tired you really are.

You are proud of the staff and how they handled each aspect of the event. You will be eager to praise them.

In the fact phase, share any of the information provided above.

In the thought phase, share the following information: You could have been killed.

In the reaction phase, share the following information: You felt helpless when he pulled the gun and made you walk through the building

In the symptom phase, share the following information: You wanted to be hugged by your spouse and children repeatedly all evening. You called your parents and siblings to talk with them, something you rarely do. (Maybe being closer to your family is a *good* outcome!)

Scenario C.1

Father Seeking Child

Vice Principal

THE INCIDENT:

Yesterday morning at 10:00 a.m., the non-custodial father of a fifth grader came into the school demanding that his son be released to him. When the principal refused to release the child or to identify his location, the father pulled out a gun and forced the principal to walk through the building to his son's classroom.

The principal stalled for time, knowing that the police had been called. When the police arrived, the father ran out of the building and began shooting back at the police. In the ensuing gun battle, the father was killed.

YOUR ROLE IN THIS INCIDENT:

You were in the office area and witnessed the whole thing. Once you saw the gun, you felt "frozen" in place. You wanted to alert the staff in the building and were able to use the intercom to instruct teachers to lock their doors and to not dismiss classes. You think you should have done more.

In the fact phase, share any of the information provided above.

In the thought phase, share the following information: While one part of you knows you did everything you could, you feel you should have done more.

In the reaction phase, share the following information: The sense of helplessness and lack of control during the event have been hard to handle.

In the symptom phase, share the following information: Your stomach was upset most of the evening and you had trouble concentrating on the TV shows you were watching.

You would secretly like a little reassurance from your co-workers.

Scenario C.1

Father Seeking Child

Secretary

THE INCIDENT:

Yesterday morning at 10:00 a.m., the non-custodial father of a fifth grader came into the school demanding that his son be released to him. When the principal refused to release the child or to identify his location, the father pulled out a gun and forced the principal to walk through the building to his son's classroom.

The principal stalled for time, knowing that the police had been called. When the police arrived, the father ran out of the building and began shooting back at the police. In the ensuing gun battle, the father was killed.

YOUR ROLE IN THIS INCIDENT:

You could see the whole scene through the office windows. You called the police when you saw him pull out the gun. It seemed to take forever for the police to arrive even though it was really only a few minutes. You were very frightened and did not know what to do about alerting the rest of the building. Everything seemed to be happening in slow motion.

In the fact phase, share any of the information provided above.

In the thought phase, share the following information: I wish I had done something more. It seems like all I did was watch.

In the reaction phase, share the following information: Your spouse wants you to quit this job and go to work someplace else. Schools are too dangerous these days.

In the symptom phase, share the following information: You keep seeing him point the gun and imagining him shooting the principal, like a slow motion instant replay on television.

Scenario C.1

Father Seeking Child

Teacher #1

THE INCIDENT:

Yesterday morning at 10:00 a.m., the non-custodial father of a fifth grader came into the school demanding that his son be released to him. When the principal refused to release the child or to identify his location, the father pulled out a gun and forced the principal to walk through the building to his son's classroom.

The principal stalled for time, knowing that the police had been called. When the police arrived, the father ran out of the building and began shooting back at the police. In the ensuing gun battle, the father was killed.

YOUR ROLE IN THIS INCIDENT:

You saw the parent enter the building. You were somewhat familiar with the situation and thought briefly about saying something to him but didn't. You went on to the staff lounge and missed the whole thing.

In the fact phase, share any of the information provided above.

In the thought phase, share the following information: What would have happened if you had stopped to talk to the parent?

In the reaction phase, share the following information: Your world has been turned upside down. If you can't be safe in a school, where can you be safe?

In the symptom phase, share the following information: You have been having intrusive mental replays of seeing the father enter the building, but then shooting at you.

Scenario C.1

Father Seeking Child

Teacher #2 (Male)

THE INCIDENT:

Yesterday morning at 10:00 a.m., the non-custodial father of a fifth grader came into the school demanding that his son be released to him. When the principal refused to release the child or to identify his location, the father pulled out a gun and forced the principal to walk through the building to his son's classroom.

The principal stalled for time, knowing that the police had been called. When the police arrived, the father ran out of the building and began shooting back at the police. In the ensuing gun battle, the father was killed.

YOUR ROLE IN THIS INCIDENT:

You are a friend of the father. You can't believe he did it. You know some of his background. He was a Vietnam veteran, had many problems due to Post Traumatic Stress Disorder (PTSD), had difficulties with alcohol, and had recently been divorced from the child's mother. You were hunting buddies and had recently been fishing together.

You knew he was having difficulties but would have never guessed that he was capable of this.

In the fact phase, share any of the information provided above.

In the thought phase, share the following information: There must have been something you could have done to prevent this incident—some clue you missed.

In the reaction phase, share the following information: You fear others will blame you or treat you differently because you are a veteran, too.

In the symptom phase, share the following information: You are having flashbacks to an event in Viet Nam, where you witnessed one of your friends being shot by another GI.

Your secret is that you'd be very relieved to hear that others don't blame you, but you don't want to ask for it.

Scenario C.1

Father Seeking Child

Teacher #3

THE INCIDENT:

Yesterday morning at 10:00 a.m., the non-custodial father of a fifth grader came into the school demanding that his son be released to him. When the principal refused to release the child or to identify his location, the father pulled out a gun and forced the principal to walk through the building to his son's classroom.

The principal stalled for time, knowing that the police had been called. When the police arrived, the father ran out of the building and began shooting back at the police. In the ensuing gun battle, the father was killed.

YOUR ROLE IN THIS INCIDENT:

You were in your classroom and had no idea anything was wrong. You heard some shouting; there was some running down the hall past your door. You looked out the window into the playground area and saw the father getting shot. You had all the children lay on the floor until the shooting ended.

In the fact phase, share any of the information provided above.

In the thought phase, share the following information: This building is not safe to work in.

In the reaction phase, share the following information: You are very angry at the father for doing this in the school and upsetting the children and the staff.

In the symptom phase, share the following information: You have had nightmares and flashbacks of seeing the father getting shot.

Scenario C.1

Father Seeking Child

Teacher #4

THE INCIDENT:

Yesterday morning at 10:00 a.m., the non-custodial father of a fifth grader came into the school demanding that his son be released to him. When the principal refused to release the child or to identify his location, the father pulled out a gun and forced the principal to walk through the building to his son's classroom.

The principal stalled for time, knowing that the police had been called. When the police arrived, the father ran out of the building and began shooting back at the police. In the ensuing gun battle, the father was killed.

YOUR ROLE IN THIS INCIDENT:

You teach the fifth grade class which includes the deceased's son. While you were not a direct part of the incident, you have had to deal with the student and class since then. Last night, you had nightmares about the father coming into the classroom and starting to shoot you and the children.

In the fact phase, share any of the information provided above.

In the thought phase, share the following information: You wonder what could have happened if he had reached your classroom.

In the reaction phase, share the following information: You are angry at the violation of your sense of personal safety. You are also troubled by the question: How are you going to re-integrate the son into the classroom?

In the symptom phase, share the following information: You notice that you are being overly protective of your own fifth-grader. You had trouble sending him to school today.

Scenario C.1

Father Seeking Child

School Social Worker

THE INCIDENT:

Yesterday morning at 10:00 a.m., the non-custodial father of a fifth grader came into the school demanding that his son be released to him. When the principal refused to release the child or to identify his location, the father pulled out a gun and forced the principal to walk through the building to his son's classroom.

The principal stalled for time, knowing that the police had been called. When the police arrived, the father ran out of the building and began shooting back at the police. In the ensuing gun battle, the father was killed.

YOUR ROLE IN THIS INCIDENT:

You were in the building at the time of the event, although you were not directly involved. You have been working with the child for the last few months. You have worked with the mother but not the father. You had heard about his violent tendencies but never thought he would do anything like this. In fact, you are aware of some other families that you think ***could*** do something like this.

In the fact phase, share any of the information provided above.

In the thought phase, share the following information: What are you going to do to help the child?

In the reaction phase, share the following information: What if it happens again?

In the symptom phase, share the following information: You have spent most of the night on the Internet looking for articles about how to handle kids after a crisis.

Scenario C.1

Father Seeking Child

Male Physical Education Teacher

THE INCIDENT:

Yesterday morning at 10:00 a.m., the non-custodial father of a fifth grader came into the school demanding that his son be released to him. When the principal refused to release the child or to identify his location, the father pulled out a gun and forced the principal to walk through the building to his son's classroom.

The principal stalled for time, knowing that the police had been called. When the police arrived, the father ran out of the building and began shooting back at the police. In the ensuing gun battle, the father was killed.

YOUR ROLE IN THIS INCIDENT:

You were just entering the hallway as you became aware of the heated discussion going on in front of the office. At first you didn't realize what was going on, but as you got within six feet, you saw the parent pull out a gun and demand that the principal take him to his son.

For a split second, you thought about rushing him to get the gun hand but you did not. You just stopped and tried to figure out where you could go if he started shooting.

In the fact phase, share any of the information provided above.

In the thought phase, share the following information: You could have been shot.

In the reaction phase, share the following information: You worry about what the principal thinks about what you did (or did not do). You think you should have done something. You secretly wonder if your co-workers might be blaming you for your inaction.

Scenario C.2

Father Seeking Child

Supplemental Team Assignments

THE INCIDENT:

Yesterday morning at 10:00 a.m., the non-custodial father of a fifth grader came into the school demanding that his son be released to him. When the principal refused to release the child or to identify his location, the father pulled out a gun and forced the principal to walk through the building to his son's classroom.

The principal stalled for time, knowing that the police had been called. When the police arrived, the father ran out of the building and began shooting back at the police. In the ensuing gun battle, the father was killed.

ASSIGNMENT #1

Keeping in mind the principles we have been discussing, prepare to face the media. They are waiting outside your door to talk with you. They want to bring their cameras in and want to know what students and staff they can talk to.

- Outline points to be covered by the spokesperson.
- Specify what instructions will be given to staff (per any existing crisis plan) to guide them in dealing with the media.
- What do you need to say to the parents of your students at this moment?
- Who should be consulted for approval before information is released?

ASSIGNMENT #2

- Identify any target groups to which you wish to provide immediate crisis services before they leave the building today.

ASSIGNMENT #3

What are your recommendations regarding:

- How to connect students with parents?
- What to do during the rest of the day?

ASSIGNMENT #4

- Identify the "ripple effect" of groups for which you know you will plan formal debriefings/services today.
- Predict how many staff you will need to accomplish your tasks.

ASSIGNMENT #5:

- You have been asked to give some ideas on ways to help principals in other nearby schools help their students deal with the fears engendered by this event.
- Write down some ideas for age-appropriate activities that could be done.

Father Seeking Child

Supplemental Team Assignments (Continued)

THE INCIDENT:

Yesterday morning at 10:00 a.m., the non-custodial father of a fifth grader came into the school demanding that his son be released to him. When the principal refused to release the child or to identify his location, the father pulled out a gun and forced the principal to walk through the building to his son's classroom.

The principal stalled for time, knowing that the police had been called. When the police arrived, the father ran out of the building and began shooting back at the police. In the ensuing gun battle, the father was killed.

ASSIGNMENT #6:

- What can the school staff do for parents and for the community?

ASSIGNMENT #7:

- Write some simple guidelines to help school staff to identify students who may need special attention or referral to a professional.
- What steps should be taken before making such a recommendation?

Scenario C.3

School Boiler Explosion

Facilitator's Guide Sheet

THE INCIDENT:

Two days ago at 10:00 a.m., there was a gas explosion in the boiler room of your school. A janitor was killed instantly. The explosion blew out the windows in virtually all the rooms on the west side of the building, spraying glass over dozens of children and several teachers in the playground area. Many have been transported to local hospitals and urgent care centers. The building and playground area looked like they had been hit with a bomb.

Inside the building, several staff members were severely injured. The physical education teacher (also a popular football coach) was burned so badly that he was airlifted to the burn unit of a university hospital. Miraculously, the only fatality has been the janitor. There will certainly be some scars and maybe even some lasting disabilities, but it looks like everyone else will survive.

For the last two days, the School Response Team has been working with students. All students are attending a shortened schedule at a nearby church where ample space makes it possible to continue to have school daily. They have provided you with lots of support and materials to help the kids. This is the first opportunity you have had to meet with your colleagues to talk about your own "stuff."

It is now Friday afternoon and this is a debriefing of the key staff members who the principal has "strongly encouraged" to attend. There really was no resistance.

PLACE: McClellan Elementary School

TIME: Two days ago

PERSONNEL INVOLVED:	THEME:	SYMPTOMS:
1. Principal	Still trying to regain control	No appetite; can't stop or relax
2. Vice principal	Overwhelmed; wants control	Anticipatory anxiety
3. Secretary	Loss of personal safety; sad	Anxiety attacks
4. Social worker	Feeling inadequate	Sleep disturbances
5. Teacher #1	Loss of sense of safety	Flashbacks; tremors
6. Teacher #2	Flashbacks to combat	Intrusive visual memories
7. Teacher #3	Loss of sense of safety	Over-protective of kids
8. Teacher #4	Self-doubt over actions	Nightmares; flashbacks
9. Teacher #5	Loss of sense of safety	Confusion; sensory imprinting

POSSIBLE PROCESS QUESTIONS:

- Which people needed reassurance? Did they get it? How?
- How did the issue of loss of personal safety get expressed and dealt with?
- Summarize a few good pieces of advice or teaching about managing flashbacks and nightmares.
- What were some of the good coping responses shared by the participants?
- What comments or questions could the CISM team make to facilitate more discussion of positive coping outcomes?

Scenario C.4

Teacher Car Crash

Facilitator's Guide Sheet

THE INCIDENT:

A phone call was received from the county sheriff's office that two teachers, Stan and Mary, were killed in an auto accident yesterday morning on the way to school. It was a car/deer accident on a rural two-lane highway and it appears that no one was at fault.

The car was severely damaged and Stan was thrown from the vehicle. Stan had taught at this school for over 10 years. He was one of the coaches for the softball team and was well liked by everyone. He had a great sense of humor and was quite playful.

Mary was fairly new to the area. She was somewhat quiet and not as well-known, but was accepted and respected by the staff.

A few minutes after the accident, a school bus loaded with children drove past the scene and some of the students recognized the victims.

PLACE: Grant Middle School

TIME: Yesterday: 7:30 a.m.

PERSONNEL INVOLVED:	THEME:	SYMPTOMS:
1. Friend who had an argument	Guilt	Irritable; anxious
2. Basketball and hunting friend	Shock and denial	Intrusive images
3. School secretary	Anger at rumors	Trouble concentrating
4. Friend of Mary	Thoughts of mortality	Sleep disturbance
5. Friend who turned down Mary for a ride	Guilt	Disturbing dreams
6. Stan's co-coach	What to tell kids?	Memory problems
7. Student teacher	None	None

POSSIBLE PROCESS QUESTIONS:

- What things did the CISM team do or say to help participants make connections (e.g., did anyone offer advice or company to the student teacher)?
- Did the people who needed help dealing with guilt get it? How?
- How did the team do with summarizing and addressing the various symptoms?
- Were there positive coping tips about dealing with grief? Anger? Guilt?
- Is regret and self-recrimination always a theme with grief? (YES)
- Did the issue of anger at rumors get handled? How?
- Was the team able to facilitate any lighter story-telling or eulogizing?

NOTE: *A practice debriefing for the death(s) of a colleague should be performed with care. Make sure that you have explained the event and asked participants if they have actually experienced such an event before continuing. Those individuals should be excluded from the actual role play. Even a role play of a made-up event can trigger powerful grief issues.*

Scenario C.5

Teacher Car Crash

Supplemental Team Assignments

THE INCIDENT:

A phone call was received from the county sheriff's office that two teachers, Stan and Mary, were killed in an auto accident yesterday morning on the way to school. It was a car/deer accident on a rural two-lane highway and it appears that no one was at fault.

The car was severely damaged and Stan was thrown from the vehicle. Stan had taught at this school for over 10 years. He was one of the coaches for the softball team and was well liked by everyone. He had a great sense of humor and was quite playful.

Mary was fairly new to the area. She was somewhat quiet and not as well-known, but was accepted and respected by the staff.

A few minutes after the accident, a school bus loaded with children drove past the scene and some of the students recognized the victims.

ASSIGNMENT #1:

- Outline points to be covered by the spokesperson
- Specify what instructions will be given to staff (per any existing crisis plan) to guide them in any dealings with the media
- What should be said to parents of students at this moment?
- Who should be consulted for approval before information is released?

ASSIGNMENT #2:

- Identify any target groups to which you wish to provide immediate crisis services before they leave the building today.

ASSIGNMENT #3:

What are your recommendations regarding:

- How to connect students with parents?
- What to do during the rest of the day?

ASSIGNMENT #4:

- Identify the "ripple effect" of groups for which you know you will plan formal debriefings/services tomorrow.
- Predict how many staff you need to accomplish your tasks.

Teacher Car Crash

Supplemental Team Assignments (continued)

THE INCIDENT:

A phone call was received from the county sheriff's office that two teachers, Stan and Mary, were killed in an auto accident yesterday morning on the way to school. It was a car/deer accident on a rural two-lane highway and it appears that no one was at fault.

The car was severely damaged and Stan was thrown from the vehicle. Stan had taught at this school for over 10 years. He was one of the coaches for the softball team and was well liked by everyone. He had a great sense of humor and was quite playful.

Mary was fairly new to the area. She was somewhat quiet and not as well-known, but was accepted and respected by the staff.

A few minutes after the accident, a school bus loaded with children drove past the scene and some of the students recognized the victims.

ASSIGNMENT #5:

- You have been asked to give some ideas on ways to help principals in other nearby schools to help their students deal with the fears engendered by this event.
- Write down some ideas for age appropriate activities that could be done.

ASSIGNMENT #6:

- What can the school staff do for parents and the community?

ASSIGNMENT #7:

- Write some simple guidelines to help school staff identify students who may need special attention or referral to a professional.
- What steps should be taken before making such a recommendation?

Scenario C.6

Teacher Suicide

Facilitator's Guide Sheet

THE INCIDENT:

School personnel were shocked to learn about the death of Joe, a teacher for 12 years. Joe hanged himself at some point during the night.

Within the last six weeks, his wife had left him, and he had been increasingly depressed. He had been drinking more lately, although few people were aware of it. The night before last, Joe went out to a bar with two staff members. They had some drinks and eventually left him there.

Yesterday morning when he didn't show up for his regular carpool and breakfast, the other teachers thought he had just gone to school early. After arriving at the school and discovering that Joe had not shown up, two friends were sent to Joe's house where they found the front door unlocked and Joe hanging in his bedroom. There was no suicide note.

It is now 24 hours later.

PLACE: Buell High School

TIME: Yesterday: 7:30 a.m.

PERSONNEL INVOLVED:	THEME:	SYMPTOMS:
1. Joe's confidant	Anger/guilt	Confusion/sadness
2. Jazz buddy	Sorrow	Loss of interest
3. Drinking buddy #1	Guilt	Intrusive thoughts
4. Drinking buddy #2	Guilt	Poor sleep; concentration
5. Friend #1 who found the body	Conflicting sad/mad	Visual images/dreams
6. Friend #2 who found the body	Guilt	Visual images
7. Friend #3	Shaken beliefs	Lost appetite
8. Student teacher	Compassion	None

POSSIBLE PROCESS QUESTIONS:

- Were the participants able to help each other deal with guilt and anger?
- Name some things the team did to address anger and guilt (e.g., was "refragmentation" necessary)?
- How did this suicide shake the beliefs of the various participants?

***NOTE:** A practice debriefing for the death(s) of a colleague should be performed with care. Make sure that you have explained the event and asked participants if they have actually experienced such an event before continuing. Those who have should be excluded from the actual role play. Even a role play of a made-up event can trigger powerful grief issues.*

Scenario C.7

Student Death at Football Game

Facilitator's Guide Sheet

THE INCIDENT:

Last Friday night a popular high school senior, Danny Smith, fell from the top row of the stands during a football game. He had been drinking alcohol with several friends prior to and during the game and had a fight with his girlfriend earlier in the evening. He had been sitting on the top row of the stands when he suddenly stood up and tried to sit on the top rail. He lost his balance and fell to his death.

Five or six students were nearby and clearly witnessed the event. Another dozen or so surrounded the body until the ambulance crew was able to get there and eventually remove him. He died at the hospital later in the evening.

During the day, the School Response Team has been working with students. They have provided a lot of support and materials to help the kids. This is the first opportunity you have had to meet with your colleagues to talk about your own "stuff."

It is now Monday afternoon and this is a debriefing of the key staff members who the principal has "strongly encouraged" to attend. There was no resistance to attending the debriefing.

PLACE: Arnold High School

TIME: Three days ago

PERSONNEL INVOLVED:	THEME:	SYMPTOMS:
1. Vice principal	Guilt feelings	Trouble sleeping
2. Drama teacher	Guilt	Flashbacks to previous
3. Teacher	Feeling of helplessness	Overprotection of sons
4. Guidance counselor	Guilt; helpless; hopeless	Depression
5. Swim coach	Helpless; talk to parents	Sleeping; brother's death
6. Father's friend	Feeling inadequate	Protective of son
7. Teacher/parent	Guilt; fear for son	Crying; fear for son
8. Mother's friend	Numb	Difficult concentrating

POSSIBLE PROCESS QUESTIONS:

- Which people needed reassurance? Did they get it? How?
- How did the issue of loss of personal safety get expressed and dealt with?
- Summarize a few good pieces of advice or teaching about managing flashbacks and nightmares.
- What were some of the good coping responses shared by the participants?
- What comments or questions could the CISM team make to facilitate more discussion of positive coping outcomes?

Scenario C.8

Former Student Takes Hostages

Facilitator's Guide Sheet

THE INCIDENT:

A 14-year-old male entered the school by the front door carrying a large gym bag as he walked purposefully down the hall. He was seen, but ignored, by two teachers before being confronted by the assistant principal. The young man pulled a semi-automatic weapon from the bag, pointed it at the assistant principal, and then ran into an 8th-grade classroom where he took the class and the teacher (Miss Nelson) hostage.

The assistant principal ran into the office telling a secretary to call 911. They heard shots fired. The principal then ran to Miss Nelson's room and found it locked and shaded. He/she began to evacuate adjoining rooms, instructing teachers to walk students to the neighboring high school. More shots were heard and chaos spread through the hallways. The principal gave evacuation instructions to the rest of the school over the PA system.

In Miss Nelson's room, the perpetrator pointed the gun at the teacher and children. Miss Nelson confronted him by asking for the gun. He shot her once in the shoulder. She fell and was cared for by two students who applied pressure to her wound. At the end of an hour, he surrendered with no further violence. Miss Nelson was taken to the hospital where she is now in fair condition after surgery. The shooter was later identified by the teacher he passed in the hallway as Johnnie Jones, a former student who was expelled.

PLACE: McKinley Junior High School (7th and 8th grades)

TIME: Yesterday: 9:00 a.m.

PERSONNEL INVOLVED:	THEME:	SYMPTOMS:
1. Principal	Worrying about others	Much closer to family
2. Assistant principal	Thoughts of mortality	Not eating
3. School secretary	Helpless; slow motion	Spouse wants her to quit
4. Teacher in hall #1	Second-guessing self	Poor concentration
5. Teacher in hall #2	Anger at media	Trouble sleeping
6. Co-teacher #3	Loss of safety	Nightmares; flashbacks
7. Co-teacher #4	Grateful to social worker	Anger
8. School social worker	Worries about adequacy	Depression; no energy
9. Teacher #5	Worries about adequacy	Indigestion
10. Teacher #6	Grief/loss of sister	Crying

POSSIBLE PROCESS QUESTIONS:

- Which people needed reassurance? Did they get it? How?
- How did the issue of loss of personal safety get expressed and dealt with?
- Summarize a few good pieces of advice or teaching about managing flashbacks and nightmares.
- What were some of the good coping responses shared by the participants?
- What comments or questions could the CISM team make to facilitate more discussion of positive coping outcomes?

Scenario C.9

Father Shoots Vice Principal

Facilitator's Guide Sheet

THE INCIDENT:

At noon yesterday, the father of one of the school's students entered the building. Going directly to the administrative area, he pushed past the secretary and went into the office where he pulled a gun and shot Vice Principal Herb Smedlap three times.

The father then left the area to go outside and wait for the police to arrive. He was arrested about 10 minutes after the incident.

The man's son, Jimmy Jones, had been a disciplinary problem for many years and the family had several confrontations with the staff in the past. The father apparently was angry over the most recent disciplinary action taken against his son. Jimmy had been sent to the office for a minor infraction of the rules. If it had been anyone but Jimmy, the situation might have been ignored.

Herb is in critical condition at the local hospital. It is unknown at the present time if he will survive. There is some speculation that if he does live, he may be paralyzed from the waist down.

Since the shooting took place during the lunch period, chaos reigned for quite some time. Rumors were flying, kids were out of control in the hallways, and it was very difficult for staff to find out what had happened and determine what they should so.

PLACE: Berry Creek Middle School

TIME: Yesterday: Noon

PERSONNEL INVOLVED:	THEME:	SYMPTOMS:
1. School secretary	Helpless; flashbacks	Anxiety; physical symptoms
2. Teacher #1	Guilt about the discipline	Panic attacks
3. Teacher #2	Guilt about not talking to father	Withdrawal
4. Teacher #3	Why Herb?	Feeling overwhelmed
5. School janitor	Guilt	Flashbacks
6. School counselor	Guilt	Feeling locked up
7. Wrestling coach	Guilt	Hypervigilant

POSSIBLE PROCESS QUESTIONS:

- Which people needed reassurance? Did they get it?
- How did the team help this process? What could they have done differently?
- How did the issue of guilt get expressed and dealt with?
- Summarize a few good pieces of advice or teaching about managing guilt.
- What comments or questions could the CISM team make to facilitate more discussion of positive coping outcomes?

COMMUNITY-BASED EXPERIENCES

Scenario D.1

Bank Robbery

Facilitator's Guide Sheet

THE INCIDENT:

At 2:45 yesterday an individual entered the bank on South Main Street and waited in line for the next available teller. When his turn came, he approached the teller and presented a note that read, "This is a robbery. I have a gun. Put all the money in a bag. Don't put in a dye packet. And don't touch the alarm button."

The teller took out a bag and started filling it with bills from the drawer, leaving the larger notes. The teller tried to get the attention of other tellers so that they could sound the alarm, but all the other tellers were busy with customers.

After the teller handed the man the bag, he fled out the door. The teller pushed the alarm and shouted that a man had just robbed the bank.

A teller, who was returning from a meeting downtown, saw the fleeing robber and followed him to the parking lot where the teller obtained the license number of his vehicle. The teller returned to the bank and added this information to that already telephoned to the police.

The police arrived and began interviewing the tellers, staff, and bank patrons. About 20 minutes later, the police reported to the tellers that they had just received word that another unit had stopped the suspect's car, found the bank bag under the front seat, and arrested the suspect.

PLACE: Green River National Bank

TIME: Three Days Ago: 2:45 p.m.

PERSONNEL INVOLVED:	THEME:	SYMPTOMS:
1. Teller #1 who was robbed	Frustration vs. fear	Delayed response; easily startled
2. Teller #2 at the next window	Has history	Fear of repetition; anxiety; dreams
3. Teller #3 returning from meeting	Pleased with self	None; feels stronger
4. Teller #4 at the drive through	Helpless	Sleep; avoidance; irritable
5. Branch manager	Helpless; anger	Overprotective

POSSIBLE PROCESS QUESTIONS:

- Who were the people needing reassurance? Did they get it? How?
- How did the issue of loss of personal safety get expressed and dealt with?
- Summarize a few good pieces of advice or teaching about managing flashbacks and nightmares.
- What were some of the good coping responses shared by the participants?
- What comments or questions could the CISM team make to facilitate more discussion of positive coping outcomes?

Scenario D.1

Bank Robbery

Overview

THE INCIDENT:

At 2:45 yesterday an individual entered the bank on South Main Street and waited in line for the next available teller. When his turn came, he approached the teller and presented a note that read, "This is a robbery. I have a gun. Put all the money in a bag. Don't put in a dye packet. And don't touch the alarm button."

The teller took out a bag and started filling it with bills from the drawer, leaving the larger notes. The teller tried to get the attention of other tellers so that they could sound the alarm, but all the other tellers were busy with customers.

After the teller handed the man the bag, he fled out the door. The teller pushed the alarm and shouted that a man had just robbed the bank.

A teller, who was returning from a meeting downtown, saw the fleeing robber and followed him to the parking lot where the teller obtained the license number of his vehicle. The teller returned to the bank and added this information to that already telephoned to the police.

The police arrived and began interviewing the tellers, staff, and bank patrons. About 20 minutes later, the police reported to the tellers that they had just received word that another unit had stopped the suspect's car, found the bank bag under the front seat, and arrested the suspect.

PLACE: Green River National Bank

TIME: Three Days Ago: 2:45 p.m.

PERSONNEL INVOLVED:

1. Teller #1 who was robbed
2. Teller #2 at the next window
3. Teller #3 returning from meeting
4. Teller #4 at the drive through
5. Branch manager

Scenario D.1

Bank Robbery

Teller #1 Who Was Robbed

THE INCIDENT:

At 2:45 yesterday an individual entered the bank on South Main Street and waited in line for the next available teller. When his turn came, he approached the teller and presented a note that read, "This is a robbery. I have a gun. Put all the money in a bag. Don't put in a dye packet. And don't touch the alarm button."

The teller took out a bag and started filling it with bills from the drawer, leaving the larger notes. The teller tried to get the attention of other tellers so that they could sound the alarm, but all the other tellers were busy with customers.

After the teller handed the man the bag, he fled out the door. The teller pushed the alarm and shouted that a man had just robbed the bank.

A teller, who was returning from a meeting downtown, saw the fleeing robber and followed him to the parking lot where the teller obtained the license number of his vehicle. The teller returned to the bank and added this information to that already telephoned to the police.

The police arrived and began interviewing the tellers, staff, and bank patrons. About 20 minutes later, the police reported to the tellers that they had just received word that another unit had stopped the suspect's car, found the bank bag under the front seat, and arrested the suspect.

YOUR ROLE IN THIS INCIDENT:

You are the teller who was robbed.

In the fact phase, share any of the information provided above.

In the thought phase, share the following information: Your first thought was of the bank robbery that had occurred at your branch three months ago. You know that no one was arrested in that robbery. You also thought that the man had a gun and that he would have shot you if you didn't follow his directions.

In the reaction phase, share the following information: You are angry that the robber put you, your fellow employees, and the bank patrons in jeopardy. You remember thinking a mile-a-minute, "What if I could..." and you remember being very frustrated that you couldn't make eye contact with anyone, but also being afraid. It wasn't until after the event that you became shaky and found it difficult to concentrate on the questions the police were asking.

In the symptom phase, share the following information: Since this event took place, you have continued to work but you worry about the possibility of being robbed even by regular bank patrons. Yesterday, one of your regular customers handed you a note and you nearly pushed the alarm. The note simply indicated how sorry she was to read about the robbery and how she hoped you were doing well. You are pleased that the police caught the suspect, but you know that you will probably have to go to court to testify. Your spouse has been supportive and things have been a little better today.

Scenario D.1

Bank Robbery

Teller #2 At The Next Window

THE INCIDENT:

At 2:45 yesterday an individual entered the bank on South Main Street and waited in line for the next available teller. When his turn came, he approached the teller and presented a note that read, "This is a robbery. I have a gun. Put all the money in a bag. Don't put in a dye packet. And don't touch the alarm button."

The teller took out a bag and started filling it with bills from the drawer, leaving the larger notes. The teller tried to get the attention of other tellers so that they could sound the alarm, but all the other tellers were busy with customers.

After the teller handed the man the bag, he fled out the door. The teller pushed the alarm and shouted that a man had just robbed the bank.

A teller, who was returning from a meeting downtown, saw the fleeing robber and followed him to the parking lot where the teller obtained the license number of his vehicle. The teller returned to the bank and added this information to that already telephoned to the police.

The police arrived and began interviewing the tellers, staff, and bank patrons. About 20 minutes later, the police reported to the tellers that they had just received word that another unit had stopped the suspect's car, found the bank bag under the front seat, and arrested the suspect.

YOUR ROLE IN THIS INCIDENT:

You are the teller who was at the window next to the teller who was robbed. You were busy with an older customer all the time the robber was in the bank.

In the fact phase, share any of the information provided above.

In the thought phase, share the following information: When your friend yelled that the bank had been robbed, your customer panicked, and you were afraid that she was going to faint. You are the teller who was robbed three months ago and that entire scene flashed back in your mind.

In the reaction phase, share the following information: You know what a lonely feeling it is when the robber is watching your every move and you regret that you couldn't help your friend. You usually exchange glances with all the other tellers throughout the day and if you hadn't been so occupied with the elderly patron, you would have noticed that your friend was trying to get you to sound the alarm.

In the symptom phase, share the following information: You are certain that this is not the same robber who robbed you, but you keep dreaming that the first robber is coming back again. Since this second robbery, you wake up sweating and having difficulty breathing. You want to be there for the teller who was robbed, but you are not sure that you are strong enough.

Scenario D.1

Bank Robbery

Teller #3 Returning From Meeting

THE INCIDENT:

At 2:45 yesterday an individual entered the bank on South Main Street and waited in line for the next available teller. When his turn came, he approached the teller and presented a note that read, "This is a robbery. I have a gun. Put all the money in a bag. Don't put in a dye packet. And don't touch the alarm button."

The teller took out a bag and started filling it with bills from the drawer, leaving the larger notes. The teller tried to get the attention of other tellers so that they could sound the alarm, but all the other tellers were busy with customers.

After the teller handed the man the bag, he fled out the door. The teller pushed the alarm and shouted that a man had just robbed the bank.

A teller, who was returning from a meeting downtown, saw the fleeing robber and followed him to the parking lot where the teller obtained the license number of his vehicle. The teller returned to the bank and added this information to that already telephoned to the police.

The police arrived and began interviewing the tellers, staff, and bank patrons. About 20 minutes later, the police reported to the tellers that they had just received word that another unit had stopped the suspect's car, found the bank bag under the front seat, and arrested the suspect.

YOUR ROLE IN THIS INCIDENT:

You had just returned to the branch from a meeting downtown when you saw the man exiting through the main entrance. You followed him to the parking lot and obtained the license plate number of his vehicle. You then returned to the bank and told the police.

In the fact phase, share any of the information provided above.

In the thought phase, share the following information: You remembered vividly the meeting after the last bank robbery and knew that employees should be observant but not put themselves in danger. You noted the robber's height as he passed by the markings at the door and mentally noted the clothing he was wearing. It appeared to you that he thought you were a bank patron and didn't even look around when you followed him out of the bank. Your first thought was to nail this guy if you could. You were pleased when you were able to get the license plate number of the car.

In the reaction phase, share the following information: You work hard for your money and you are tired of these dead beats coming into the bank and robbing it. You have been angry and scared, but now feel calmer and more confident again.

In the symptom phase, share the following information: Like the other tellers, you have had flashbacks of the previous robbery in which they didn't catch anyone. You feel a lot better because the police made an arrest in this case. Your spouse suggested that you request a transfer to another branch, but you like working with your fellow employees at this branch. You know that together the crew will get through this.You are really feeling more confident than ever.

Scenario D.1

Bank Robbery

Teller #4 At The Drive Through Window

THE INCIDENT:

At 2:45 yesterday an individual entered the bank on South Main Street and waited in line for the next available teller. When his turn came, he approached the teller and presented a note that read, "This is a robbery. I have a gun. Put all the money in a bag. Don't put in a dye packet. And don't touch the alarm button."

The teller took out a bag and started filling it with bills from the drawer, leaving the larger notes. The teller tried to get the attention of other tellers so that they could sound the alarm, but all the other tellers were busy with customers.

After the teller handed the man the bag, he fled out the door. The teller pushed the alarm and shouted that a man had just robbed the bank.

A teller, who was returning from a meeting downtown, saw the fleeing robber and followed him to the parking lot where the teller obtained the license number of his vehicle. The teller returned to the bank and added this information to that already telephoned to the police.

The police arrived and began interviewing the tellers, staff, and bank patrons. About 20 minutes later, the police reported to the tellers that they had just received word that another unit had stopped the suspect's car, found the bank bag under the front seat, and arrested the suspect.

YOUR ROLE IN THIS INCIDENT:

You observed the robber through your drive through window going to his car. You then saw the teller returning from downtown following him.

In the fact phase, share any of the information provided above.

In the thought phase, share the following information: You were afraid that the robber would discover the teller who was following him. You also knew that you had to try to get a good description of the robber.

In the reaction phase, share the following information: You were protected behind that bulletproof window, but you knew that if the robber discovered the teller following him that she might be shot and you knew that you couldn't watch.

In the symptom phase, share the following information: You have replayed the entire scene over several times in the last three days. You have had difficulty sleeping and have been irritable to your family and friends because they want you to talk about it.

Scenario D.1

Bank Robbery

Branch Manager

THE INCIDENT:

At 2:45 yesterday an individual entered the bank on South Main Street and waited in line for the next available teller. When his turn came, he approached the teller and presented a note that read, "This is a robbery. I have a gun. Put all the money in a bag. Don't put in a dye packet. And don't touch the alarm button."

The teller took out a bag and started filling it with bills from the drawer, leaving the larger notes. The teller tried to get the attention of other tellers so that they could sound the alarm, but all the other tellers were busy with customers.

After the teller handed the man the bag, he fled out the door. The teller pushed the alarm and shouted that a man had just robbed the bank.

A teller, who was returning from a meeting downtown, saw the fleeing robber and followed him to the parking lot where the teller obtained the license number of his vehicle. The teller returned to the bank and added this information to that already telephoned to the police.

The police arrived and began interviewing the tellers, staff, and bank patrons. About 20 minutes later, the police reported to the tellers that they had just received word that another unit had stopped the suspect's car, found the bank bag under the front seat, and arrested the suspect.

YOUR ROLE IN THIS INCIDENT:

You were in your office with a bank patron when you heard the alarm go off.

In the fact phase, share any of the information provided above.

In the thought phase, share the following information: Your first thought was for the employees. You remember from the training after the last robbery how important it is to keep calm and to try to control the situation.

In the reaction phase, share the following information: You are angry at the robber and what his actions did to the employees at the branch.

In the symptom phase, share the following information: You don't want to leave the office for lunch or other meetings because you are afraid there will be another robbery.

Scenario D.2

Staff Car Crash

Facilitator's Guide Sheet

THE INCIDENT:

A phone call was received from the county sheriff's office that two persons, Stan and Mary, were killed in an auto accident yesterday morning on the way to school. It was a car/deer accident on a rural two-lane highway and it appears that no one was at fault.

The car was severely damaged and Stan was thrown from the vehicle. Stan had been employed at the company for over 10 years. He was well liked by the other employees and had a great sense of humor. He was also one of the coaches for a local little league team.

Mary was fairly new to the company. She was somewhat quiet and not as well-known, but was accepted and respected by the staff.

PLACE: Quick Grow Fertilizer Company

TIME: Yesterday: 7:30 a.m.

PERSONNEL INVOLVED:

1. Friend who argued with Stan
2. Basketball and hunting friend
3. Receptionist
4. Friend of Mary
5. Friend who turned down Mary for a ride
6. Stan's friend and co-coach
7. New employee

THEME:

Guilt
Shock and denial
Anger at rumors
Thoughts of mortality
Guilt

What to tell kids?
Fear of funteral

SYMPTOMS:

Irritable; anxious
Intrusive images
Trouble concentrating
Sleep disturbance
Disturbing dreams

Memory problems
Sadness

POSSIBLE PROCESS QUESTIONS:

- Did the people who needed help dealing with guilt get it? How?
- What things did the CISM team do or say to help participants make connections (e.g., did anyone offer advice or company to the new employee)?
- How did the team do with summarizing and addressing the various symptoms?
- Is regret and self-recrimination always a theme with grief? (YES)
- Did the issue of anger at rumors get handled? How?

NOTE: *A practice debriefing for the death(s) of a colleague should be performed with care. Make sure that you have explained the event and asked participants if they have actually experienced such an event before continuing. Those individuals should be excluded from the actual role play. Even a role play of a made-up event can trigger powerful grief issues.*

Scenario D.3

Staff Car Crash

Supplemental Team Assignments

THE INCIDENT:

A phone call was received from the county sheriff's office that two persons, Stan and Mary, were killed in an auto accident yesterday morning on the way to school. It was a car/deer accident on a rural two-lane highway and it appears that no one was at fault.

The car was severely damaged and Stan was thrown from the vehicle. Stan had been employed at the company for over 10 years. He was well liked by the other employees and had a great sense of humor. He was also one of the coaches for a local little league team.

Mary was fairly new to the company. She was somewhat quiet and not as well-known, but was accepted and respected by the staff.

ASSIGNMENT #1

Keeping in mind the principles we have discussed, prepare to face the media. They are waiting outside your door to talk with you. They want to bring their cameras in and want to know what staff they can talk to.)

- Outline points to be covered by the spokesperson.
- Specify what instructions will be given to staff to guide them in any dealings with the media.
- What do you need to say to the families of your staff at this moment?
- Who should be consulted for approval before information is released?

ASSIGNMENT #2

- How would you identify any target groups to which you wish to provide immediate crisis services before they leave the building today?
- What questions would need to be asked?

ASSIGNMENT #3

What are your recommendations regarding:

- What to do during the rest of the day?
- What do you suggest should be done tomorrow?
- How should the business operate?

ASSIGNMENT #4

- What can the business do for the families?

ASSIGNMENT #5

- Write some simple guidelines to help management identify personnel who may need special attention or referral to a professional.
- What steps should be taken before making such a referral?

Scenario D.4

Church Deacon Suicide

Facilitator's Guide Sheet

THE INCIDENT:

A church with a staff of 10 was shocked to learn about the death of Joe, a deacon for 12 years. Deacon Joe hanged himself at some point during the night.

Within the last six weeks, his had wife left him, he had been increasingly depressed, and had been drinking more lately—although few people were aware of it.

The night before last, Joe went out to a bar with two of the staff. They had some drinks and eventually left him there.

Yesterday morning when he didn't show up for his regular breakfast and ride to a meeting, the other deacon thought he had just gone on to the meeting early. After arriving at the meeting and discovering that Joe had not shown up, he and a co-worker were sent to Joe's house where they found the front door unlocked and Joe hanging in his bedroom. There was no suicide note.

It is now 24 hours later.

PLACE: Main Street Church

TIME: Yesterday: 7:30 a.m.

PERSONNEL INVOLVED:	THEME:	SYMPTOMS:
1. Joe's best friend	Anger/guilt	Confusion/sadness
2. Jazz buddy	Sorrow	Loss of interest
3. Drinking buddy #1	Guilt	Intrusive thoughts
4. Drinking buddy #2	Guilt	Poor sleep; concentration
5. Friend #3 who found the body	Conflicting sad and mad	Visual images/dreams
6. Friend #4 who found the body	Guilt	Visual images
7. Friend #5	Shaken beliefs	Lost appetite
8. New staff person	Compassion	None

POSSIBLE PROCESS QUESTIONS:

- Were there special issues in this event because of the spiritual component?
- Were the spiritual issues discussed?
- Were the participants able to help each other deal with guilt and anger?
- Name some things the team did to address anger and guilt (e.g., was "refragmentation" necessary?).
- How did this suicide shake the beliefs of the various participants?

NOTE: *The role playing of a suicide death of a colleague may generate very intense reactions for some of the role players. Make sure that you have explained the event and asked participants if they have actually experienced such an event before continuing. Those individuals should be excluded from the actual role play. Even a role play of a made-up event can trigger powerful grief issues.*

Scenario D.5

Factory Worker Suicide

Facilitator's Guide Sheet

THE INCIDENT:

John, a 36-year-old male, committed suicide last Sunday morning. John was married with two sons, ages 12 and 14. He had been employed at the Fillmore Widget Factory for 16 years. Last February, John's position was eliminated in a corporate downsizing and he was placed on permanent lay-off status. For several months, he actively sought other employment without success. In March, he started drinking alcohol heavily. In September, his wife filed for divorce and told him to move out of the family home. Since the move, he had been allowed to see his two boys every other weekend.

Last weekend, John asked a friend if his boys could spend Saturday night at the friend's house with the friend's boys. In the early morning hours, John shot himself with a shotgun.

The Human Resources Director of the Fillmore Widget Factory contacted the CISM team because four current employees who had worked with John during his entire tenure with the company are experiencing difficulties with the suicide. The four men and their families had socialized with John and his family for the last 10 or 12 years. They bowled on the same league, went hunting and fishing together, and often their families would have get-togethers.

PLACE: Fillmore Widget Factory

TIME: Thursday: 9:00 a.m.

PERSONNEL INVOLVED:	THEME:	SYMPTOMS:
1. HR director	Well meaning; should not be there	None
2. Friend #1 (babysitting)	Angry at desertion	Irritable; isolating self
3. Friend #2 (bowling)	20-20 hindsight; guilt	Preoccupied; coser to family
4. Friend #3 (CD player)	Blaming company; sad	Lacks motivation; insomnia
5. Friend #4 (shotgun)	Blaming self	Sleep disturbance
6. Confidant	Self-blame; needs assurance	Worries
7. Friend #5	Minor anger; abandonment	Irritable; moody

POSSIBLE PROCESS QUESTIONS:

- How did (should) the CISM coordinator handle the problem of the HR director being there?
- Did the theme of self-blame get handled? What were the most helpful things said?
- Did "defragmentation" get accomplished?
- How is suicide worse than other deaths?
- What good mutual support did the discussion generate?
- Name one thing you will use from this experience.

NOTE: *This scenario is designed for a two-part role play. The call from the human resources director to the CISM coordinator can be an experiement in gathering information and then doing the debriefing or defusing. The HR person doesn't belong in the response, but is told to try to include him/herself. This is meant to start discussion about the importance of the coordinator's information gathering and making decisions about the group.*

Scenario D.6

Group Home Resident Death

Facilitator's Guide Sheet

THE INCIDENT:

The event is the natural, but sudden death of a 35-year-old male resident, named Dennis, living in a group home setting. Dennis had been sick with a cold and fever for 1 to 2 days before the group home staff brought him to the hospital. He was diagnosed with pneumonia. The court-appointed guardian had signed an emergency medical directive prior to this illness. At the hospital, the doctor began treatment, including the use of a ventilator, before discussing this with the guardian. When Dennis pulled out the ventilator, the guardian refused permission to have it reinserted and stayed away from the hospital. The only medical intervention permitted was for pain relief to make Dennis as comfortable as possible. Several group home staff members were at the hospital and watched helplessly while Dennis suffered. He died 36 hours later.

PLACE: Haveman Group Home

TIME: Yesterday: noon

PERSONNEL INVOLVED:	THEME:	SYMPTOMS:
1. Direct care worker #1	Hesitant to join group	Anger; intrusive images
2. Group home director	Taking care of others	Isolated; can't concentrate
3. Program manager	Worried about $$	None
4. 3rd shift worker	Worried about job	Sleep/appetite problems
5. 2nd shift worker	"Coulda, woulda, shoulda"	Aftereffects of flu
6. Group home nurse	Pretty quiet, not too affected	Maybe some apathy
7. Support coordinator	Blaming guardian and doctor	Anger
8. Direct care worker #2	Wants to preach	Dreams
9. Direct care worker #3	Already transferred	Anger

POSSIBLE PROCESS QUESTIONS:

- Was there a problem with including any of the supervisors into this debriefing group?
- Discuss techniques for diplomatically dealing with such possible problems.
- How did the group handle possible disruptors like the "preacher"?
- What are some good ways to handle disruptive members?
- What are some good ways to handle anger in the group?
- What are some good things to say when dealing with blaming?

Scenario D.7

Meat Packing Plant Murder

Facilitator's Guide Sheet

THE INCIDENT:

Shrub Meat Packing is a small, family-owned business and Herb Smedlap was the human resources director. At noon yesterday, an employee named Jimmy Jones entered the building. Going directly to the administrative offices, he walked past several staff members without noticing them.

When he arrived in the office area, Jimmy pushed past the secretary and went into the office where he pulled a gun and shot Herb three times, killing him instantly. Jimmy then left the area to go outside, found his brother, and waited for the police to arrive. He was arrested about 10 minutes after the incident.

Jimmy was having difficulty maintaining the pace of the work he was required to do. He had been a disciplinary problem for many years and Herb had several confrontations with him in the past. Jimmy was apparently angry over the most recent disciplinary action taken, since it was a relatively minor infraction of the rules. If it had been anyone but Jimmy, the situation might have been ignored.

Since the shooting took place at lunch time, chaos reigned for quite some time. Rumors were flying, emotions were out of control and it was very difficult for staff to find out what had happened.

PLACE: Shrub Meat Packing Plant

TIME: Yesterday: noon

PERSONNEL INVOLVED:	THEME:	SYMPTOMS:
1. Herb's secretary	Loss of sense of safety	Intrusive image
2. Employee #1	Should have known	Nightmares/images
3. Employee #2	What to say to family	Wants to get drunk
4. Quality control inspector	Anger/loss of safety	Preoccupied; got lost
5. Employee #3	Guilt; helpless	Dreams
6. Jimmy's brother	Guilty; angry	Can't eat or sleep
7. Jimmy's brother's best friend	Worried	Irritable at spouse
8. Supervisor in the next office	Distracted	Sleep disturbances
9. President of the company	Guilt; self-blame	Insomnia; flashbacks

POSSIBLE PROCESS QUESTIONS:

- Did all these people belong in this group together? Who didn't?
- How did it go with the perpetrator's brother in the group? How would you have assessed whether to include or exclude him?
- Discuss ways to diplomatically deal with such possible problems.
- What are some good tips for teaching about nightmares?
- Were there any coping tips for handling alcohol abuse? Is this appropriate to talk about?
- What lessons or comments will you try to remember to use in future debriefings?

Scenario D.8

Store Hostage/Shooting

Facilitator's Guide Sheet

THE INCIDENT:

A recently-fired male entered the store by the front door carrying a large gym bag and walked purposefully down the aisle. He went into the back room where he was seen, but ignored, by two employees. When confronted by the assistant manager, the man pulled a weapon from the bag and ran into a break room where he took five employees hostage.

The manager ran into the office and told staff to call the police. Suddenly, they heard shots fired. The manager then ran back to the break room and found it locked and shaded. He/she started evacuating the building. Customers and other staff members heard the shots and became loud and afraid. Chaos spread through the aisles.

In the break room, the perpetrator pointed the gun at the staff, ordered them onto the floor and fired several shots through the windows when they did not comply fast enough. Linda Nelson confronted him and asked for the gun. He shot her once in the shoulder.

During the next hour, the gunman held the staff hostage while talking to the police outside. He occasionally pointed his weapon at the head of one of the hostages in an attempt to restore order or quiet. At the end of an hour, he surrendered with no further violence. Linda Nelson was taken to the hospital where she is in fair condition after surgery.

While everyone at the scene was in danger, the hostages are not included in this debriefing.

PLACE: Super Value Discount Groceries

TIME: Yesterday: 9:00 a.m.

PERSONNEL INVOLVED:	THEME:	SYMPTOMS:
1. Store manager	Caretaker; loss of control	Mild anxiety
2. Assistant manager	Proud, but anxious	Visual flashbacks
3. Staff person #1	Self-doubt; loss of safety	Fatigue; slight depression
4. Staff person #2 (male)	Anger; partly at media	Irritable
5. Staff person #3	Reliving old personal loss	Preoccupied
6. Staff person #4	Should have done more	Stomach problems
7. Staff person #5 (female)	Helpless anger	Irritable
8. Staff person #6	Confusion of feelings	Irritable
9. Secretary	Loss of safety	Sleep disturbance; anxiety

POSSIBLE PROCESS QUESTIONS:

- Name some specific things the CISM team said which resulted in mutual support between staff.
- Were there any unexpected themes raised? What were some of the common ones?
- What comments or information might not have been shared without this debriefing?
- Which of the participants seemed most in need of some follow-up?
- Identify a lesson or comment you'll try to remember from this experience.

Scenario D.9

Store Hostage/Shooting

Supplemental Team Assignments

THE INCIDENT:

A recently-fired male entered the store by the front door carrying a large gym bag and walked purposefully down the aisle. He went into the back room where he was seen, but ignored, by two employees. When confronted by the assistant manager, the man pulled a weapon from the bag and ran into a break room where he took five employees hostage.

The manager ran into the office and told staff to call the police. Suddenly, they heard shots fired. The manager then ran back to the break room and found it locked and shaded. He/she started evacuating the building. Customers and other staff members heard the shots and became loud and afraid. Chaos spread through the aisles.

In the break room, the perpetrator pointed the gun at the staff, ordered them onto the floor and fired several shots through the windows when they did not comply fast enough. Linda Nelson confronted him and asked for the gun. He shot her once in the shoulder.

During the next hour, the gunman held the staff hostage while talking to the police outside. He occasionally pointed his weapon at the head of one of the hostages in an attempt to restore order or quiet. At the end of an hour, he surrendered with no further violence. Linda Nelson was taken to the hospital where she is in fair condition after surgery.

While everyone at the scene was in danger, the hostages are not included in this debriefing.

ASSIGNMENT #1

Keeping in mind the principles which have been discussed, prepare to face the media:

- Outline points to be covered by the spokesperson
- Specify what instructions will be given to staff to guide them in any dealings with the media.
- What do you need to say to the families of your staff at this moment?
- Who should be consulted for approval before information is released?
- What do you need to say to customers at this moment?

ASSIGNMENT #2

You are the crisis response team called into the CEO's office to advise him/her.

- How would you identify any target groups which need immediate crisis services before they leave the building today?
- What questions need to be asked?

ASSIGNMENT #3

You are the crisis response team called into the CEO's office to advise him/her.

- What should be done during the rest of the day?
- What should be done tomorrow?
- How should the business operate?

Store Hostage/Shooting

Supplemental Team Assignments (Continued)

THE INCIDENT:

A recently-fired male entered the store by the front door carrying a large gym bag and walked purposefully down the aisle. He went into the back room where he was seen, but ignored, by two employees. When confronted by the assistant manager, the man pulled a weapon from the bag and ran into a break room where he took five employees hostage.

The manager ran into the office and told staff to call the police. Suddenly, they heard shots fired. The manager then ran back to the break room and found it locked and shaded. He/she started evacuating the building. Customers and other staff members heard the shots and became loud and afraid. Chaos spread through the aisles.

In the break room, the perpetrator pointed the gun at the staff, ordered them onto the floor and fired several shots through the windows when they did not comply fast enough. Linda Nelson confronted him and asked for the gun. He shot her once in the shoulder.

During the next hour, the gunman held the staff hostage while talking to the police outside. He occasionally pointed his weapon at the head of one of the hostages in an attempt to restore order or quiet. At the end of an hour, he surrendered with no further violence. Linda Nelson was taken to the hospital where she is in fair condition after surgery.

While everyone at the scene was in danger, the hostages are not included in this debriefing.

ASSIGNMENT 4:

You are the crisis response team called in to the CEO's office to advise him/her.

- Would you do a defusing today? On what basis did you make that decision?
- Identify the "ripple effect" of groups for which you know you will plan formal debriefing services tomorrow.
- Predict how many staff members you will need to accomplish your tasks.

ASSIGNMENT 5:

You are a group of crisis response team members. You have been asked by the CEO of the chain of stores affected by the event to give ideas for ways to help their store managers deal with the fears engendered by this event.

- Identify what information you would need to know regarding the stores most likely to be affected.
- Write down ideas for what would be appropriate activities.
- Where would you turn to get additional information or input?

ASSIGNMENT 6:

- Write some simple guidelines to help store managers identify staff who may need special attention or referral to a professional.
- Specify which steps should be taken before making that recommendation.
- Where would you go to seek additional help or information regarding this task?

SECTION 5

Group Activities

Sometimes, You Just Gotta Have Fun!

This section is divided into two parts. The first consists of four group exercises: Challenging Comments, CISM Hangman, Practicing the Introduction Phase, and Problem Debriefing Exercises. These exercises allow the educational facilitator an opportunity to provide training in a shorter format that generates energy and discussion around specific debriefing or defusing issues.

The second part of the section presents four CISM games that have been adapted from popular television quiz shows in an effort to provide training in a "fun" format. The four games, CISM Challenge, Friendly Fracas, Question Me This, and Who Wants To Be A Debriefer? require a computer with PowerPoint software and a LCD projector to be fully effective. This allows the participants and the audience to see the questions and answers at the same time.

These group activities have been designed to make learning fun and educational. The Hangman Game, for example, is a variation of the favorite children's game and can be used both to challenge and amuse while also teaching.

To add to the excitement of the group activities and games, it is a good idea to have prizes. Since there are no "losers" in these experiences, everyone should get a gag gift. We usually try to give away things that remind people not to take life too seriously. Some of our favorites are miniature police cars or fire trucks, soap bubbles, squirt guns and other playful items which can be bought at minimal expense. Remember, the point is to learn something while having fun.

All these group activities are included on the enclosed CD ROM. They can easily be modified to fit your local area or team in whatever way works for you.

Using The Group Activities

Role of the Educational Facilitator

You are in charge and responsible for making this a fun, educational, and positive experience for all involved. It sounds like a daunting task, but it really is not. It is generally true that people who are attracted to this type of work are usually willing to be nice to one another. They are interested in learning the model and being helpful, so the process usually goes very well.

If you are enthusiastic and positive in your approach, the participants will follow your lead. The most challenging part for the educational facilitator is to make sure that all feedback is presented in a positive manner. No matter how badly someone may have done, it is your responsibility to turn it into a positive learning experience. Some ways of doing this might be by saying, "I bet you will never forget to do that again!" or "Thanks for giving us a great example of how things can sometimes go wrong, and giving your team members an opportunity to practice working out of it!"

For most of the games, think of yourself as the master of ceremonies or the moderator of a TV quiz show. You are there to process the game, but also to make it fun for the participants and the audience. Don't forget to interview the contestants; it can be an opportunity to learn a little about team members. You can have the audience provide questions or you can ask them to "judge" the answers to the questions. You should make sure that they applaud the efforts of all the participants.

Getting Started

To begin, the educational facilitator must decide what is to be accomplished. It is often fun to have more "seasoned" staff be the debriefers in the Problem Debriefing exercise. They may not get "rattled" at the problems being presented, but if they are, it is okay for "newbies" to see how they get out of it (or not).

Getting Volunteers

You can be very creative in getting volunteers for the exercise. You should always explain what the game is and then ask for players. Tell them that fabulous prizes go to the team participants. For instance, if you are giving miniature police cars as one of the prizes, you can add that the winners will receive a "brand new car!"

We often handpick our "volunteers" for these experiences. This helps to break the ice and ensures participants will be comfortable with the exercise.

Each of the exercises is a team effort, so no one is singled out for pressure or embarrassment. It is the educational facilitator's job to keep the activity fun and not too personal.

Getting Organized

Once you have the participants identified, follow the instructions on the exercise. Each one is slightly different and contains a complete description. Keep the energy high and the focus on learning and fun.

Are We Ready?

Once the participants are ready, begin the process as described in the directions for each event.

Processing the Experience

The processing of the experience is usually pretty straightforward. You do a little teaching as the game goes along or you process the experience like a role-play, or you solicit feedback from the audience about other things that could have been tried. In general, try to keep the audience involved.

And, of course, have fun!

CHALLENGING COMMENTS GAME

Time: 30 to 45 minutes

Goals: Participants will learn and remember some appropriate answers to possible challenging comments often heard in a debriefing.

Materials: Enough 3x5 cards for each participant to have at least one; stop watch or timer; three sets of 3x5 cards numbered 1 to 5 for scoring; gag prizes of some sort; newsprint and easel for scorekeeper.

Procedures:

1. Divide participants into several groups:
   a Select a scorekeeper
   b. Select a group of 3 to 5 members of the audience to serve as judges; give them a set of score cards
   c. Set up two or more teams of at least 3 to 5 players

2. The audience is instructed to write on each card one comment or question that they would find difficult to respond to at a debriefing. (3 minutes).

3. (OPTIONAL) If working in small teams, the instructor can then ask each team to spend group time editing down to the three most challenging statements. (10 minutes).

4. Collect cards in such a way that each team will be asked to respond to comments written by a different team.

5. Each team is instructed to imagine being involved in a debriefing when this comment is made and give their best response. Conferring within the team is encouraged. A different team member gives the answer each time. The team has 30 seconds to respond.

6. After each response is given, the judges show their scorecards (with a number value between 1 and 5) and the scorekeeper records the total score.

7. The game progresses with teams alternating until each has had an equal number of chances and ends whenever time dictates or all questions are answered. This is generally a judgment call by the educational facilitator.

8. The scorekeeper declares the winners and the prizes are distributed.

9. The educational facilitator asks the audience for feedback. This discussion can include what made good questions and what are alternate answers to some of the particularly difficult questions. Participants are encouraged to write down some of their favorites.

HANGMAN GAME

Time: 30 minutes or longer, depending upon the number of rounds played.

Goal: This is a fun way to test the knowledge of team members regarding key concepts or phrases important in CISM work.

Materials: Newsprint: one sheet with the lines representing the word or phrase and one sheet with two "gallows" drawn on it. Gag prizes for the winners.

Procedures:

1. Divide participants into two teams.
2. Explain that the lines on the newsprint represent a word, name or phrase from CISM work. Their job is to guess letters that will eventually expose enough of the phrase so they can correctly identify it.
3. Select the team to start (flip a coin?).
4. The first team selects a letter. If the letter is in the puzzle, the facilitator places it in the correct space and the second team gets to select a letter.
5. When a letter is selected that is NOT part of the word or phrase, a body part is drawn on that team's "gallows" and the incorrect letter is placed at the bottom of the newsprint to track letters already guessed.
6. A team may guess at the phrase after the successful conclusion of placing a letter. If they guess incorrectly, another body part is added to their "gallows." The opportunity to guess the phrase then goes to the other team.
7. The first team to correctly identify the word or phrase "wins."

At this point you have a variety of options open. You can select another team to challenge the "winners" (or the losers) and play enough rounds so that everyone participates. You can also end the game and do some teaching about the word or phrase selected.

NOTE: The hangman body parts sequence is: head, body, arm, arm, leg, and leg. You can add eyes, nose, and mouth to give additional opportunities. Once a team has been "hung," they are out of the round. The other team continues until they guess correctly or are "hanged." If both teams are "hung," you can start teaching or start another round.

INTRODUCTION PHASE PRACTICE

Time: 20 to 30 minutes

Goals: Participants will practice the Introduction Phase of a debriefing or defusing, choosing appropriate introductory remarks to fit different situations.

Materials: This sheet of instructions is all you will need. Invent other example situations to fit the needs of your team.

Procedure:

1. Divide teams into small groups (6 to 8).
   a. Select three volunteers from each group to be debriefers.
   b. Give each group a role-play situation. Choose from the examples below or invent your own.
2. Each team of three debriefers withdraws to a private area to prepare their "introduction." (10 minutes)
3. Remaining group members are not expected to do much, but may want to prepare any questions they would ask in the given situation.
4. All debriefers re-join the groups. One team at a time demonstrates their "introduction" for 3 to 5 minutes each while the other groups watch.
5. Group members give feedback, discuss options, and ask questions for 3 to 5 minutes.
6. Members are encouraged to write down favorite comments or procedures.

Sample Situations:

- Defusing of an experienced fire department after a multiple child fatality fire.
- Debriefing of police inexperienced in CISD after an officer is wounded in a shoot-out.
- Debriefing school teachers inexperienced in CISD after one is killed in a bombing.
- Defusing inexperienced fire, police, and EMT's after a prolonged failed rescue.
- Debriefing police after an officer-involved shooting where procedural errors may have been made.
- Debriefing any inexperienced group that is skeptical of you.
- Debriefing an inexperienced group of employees that are forced to attend after violence in the workplace.

PROBLEM DEBRIEFING EXERCISE

Time: This exercise varies with the number of role plays done. Anticipate about 30 minutes per role play.

Goal: This exercise provides practice in responding to particularly difficult debriefing scenarios. The educational facilitator should take every opportunity for laughter (after the role plays) while paying close attention to the needs and responses of the role players.

Materials: Group instruction sheet for each group member.

Procedures:

1. Split participants into small groups of 7 to 9 and arrange them in separate circles. If the number of participants is small, you can have one group with observers.
2. Choose two debriefers from each group. These typically should be among the most experienced within the group. Ask to them step out of the room for a few minutes while the team prepares for the exercise.
3. Each group is given an instruction sheet and makes up a problem debriefing scenario, which includes enough of a description that each group member is able to play a specific role/situation. (The purpose of the scenario is to give an opportunity to practice a particularly difficult situation.)

   The educational facilitator circulates between groups to guard against too much repetition. They should give guidance to start the fact phase by saying their name and role. The debriefees should always try to give the debriefers a way to work with them and should not make things impossibly difficult.
4. The debriefers are given an outline of the debriefing they are about to conduct, without the difficult situation they will be facing. They are coached to model a good introduction and ground rules opening, to reflect the process openly, and maintain respect for the group.
5. The debriefing teams then are assigned to a group different from the one they originally came from.
6. In turn, each group then does a mini-debriefing while the rest of the group observes.
7. After an appropriate time (usually around 15 to 30 minutes), the role play is stopped by the educational facilitator and analyzed for learning purposes.
8. The remaining debriefings are completed and analyzed.

GROUP INSTRUCTIONS

In a few minutes, as realistically as possible, your group is to act out the type of problem or challenge you have chosen for your exercise. Your goal is NOT to humiliate the debriefers, but rather to give them and the audience the chance to increase their skills in handling special challenges in debriefing.

1. Make up a problem theme that your group thinks is realistic and would like to explore, or use one of the following examples.
2. Make up a critical incident scenario explaining briefly who your group is and what happened. Write it down in two or three sentences to be given to your debriefers.
3. Choose one or two volunteers to role-play the problem of the scenario. Help them think of a few things they may say or do.
4. Each of the other members should think of a role and some things they might say. These should be quickly shared with the group.
5. When your debriefers arrive, tell them your critical incident scenario, and then begin the role play.

Be kind to the debriefers by not making the role play unrealistically difficult. Remember, next time you will be in the hot seat!

Example Themes:

- Dominating group member
- Blaming someone who is not in the group
- Subgroup resistant to the debriefing and challenging it
- Administrator who is resistant or inhibiting the group
- A group member totally loses control in a way that halts the process
- One or two members try to share too much personal material (start to get into therapy issues)
- Several people express guilt, but get little or no support from their group (such as after a suicide)
- Blaming someone who is in the group (however unlikely this is to occur in reality)

CISM CHALLENGE GAME

INSTRUCTIONS FOR LOADING AND OPERATING

- Open or run PowerPoint on your computer.
- Select the file CISM CHALLENGE.PPT on the CD ROM included with this book.
- Select the slide show icon in the lower left tool bar (icon of a screen) and you will get the title screen.
- To advance to the next slide press the space bar. Each time you press the space bar, additional text or the next slide will appear. If you press the space bar too rapidly, the additional text may not project. In this case, just press the space bar again.
- When you reach the CISM CHALLENGE game board, you will find six columns with headings and five point amounts. Note that the amounts are underlined.
- To select a specific category and amount, place the cursor on the amount and depress the left mouse button.
- The answer to the question will appear. Please note the five-pointed star in the bottom right hand corner on this slide.
- To see the appropriate question, place the cursor on the five-pointed star and depress the left mouse key. When the screen appears, press the spacebar to see the appropriate question.
- To return to the game board, place the cursor on the five-pointed star and depress the left mouse key. When you return to the game board screen, you will notice that the amount of the previous question is now blank.
- Select another amount by placing the cursor on the amount and the answer of the next question will appear.
- To see the appropriate question, place the cursor on the five-pointed star and depress the left mouse key. When the screen appears, press the spacebar to see the appropriate question. Repeat this process until all amounts have been selected from the game board.

The moderator should review all the "answers" and "questions" prior to playing the game. The game is meant to reinforce teaching that has already taken place. The examples presented here may contain information that you have not already taught. You can either present this information or modify the "answers" and "questions" to material with which your participants are familiar.

The computer operator should practice several times with the program before actually playing the game so that he/she is familiar with how to operate it. It is also a good idea to have a printed copy of all the slides with the computer operator. To print a copy of the slides while the program is loaded, select "Print" from the "File" option. In the lower left hand corner there is a box that is entitled "Print What?" Select one of the options and then select how you want it printed by checking the appropriate box. Some "answers" have several lines. To project additional lines of text, the computer operator needs to depress the space bar another time. The following is a step-by-step procedure to assist you in using **CISM CHALLENGE**.

GROUP INSTRUCTIONS

- Project the first slide on the computer screen (CISM CHALLENGE).
- Select two teams of three players (or any number you wish) to play the game.
- Arrange them so that they can all see the computer screen or the projection screen.
- Select three judges to determine who raises his/her hand first when the answer is shown on the screen. All participants agree to accept the ruling of the majority of the judges on who raised his/her hand first. If you are fortunate enough to have game paddles that identify who signaled first, second, and third, then you will not need to appoint judges.
- Determine by a coin flip which team will play first.
- Project the second slide on the screen by depressing the space bar (three times for all the text to appear).
- Project the next slide by depressing the space bar (three times for all the text to appear).
- Project the game board on the screen by depressing the space bar once and describe the categories.
- The first player will select a category and a point value.
- The person operating the computer will place the cursor on the point value in the category chosen and depress the left mouse key. The category and the amount will be projected on the screen.
- The computer operator presses the space bar once and the "answer" will appear.
- The moderator will give the team 30 seconds to supply the correct question.
- After the team spokesman has answered the question, the computer operator will place the cursor on the gold star and depress the left mouse button.
- Again, a slide will appear that has the category and the amount on the top. The computer operator depresses the space bar to project the correct "question."
- To return to the game board the computer operator will place the cursor on the gold star and depress the left mouse button.
- One of the judges will mark the point value on a cumulative score sheet which is large enough for everyone to see.
- If the team correctly formed a "question" for the given "answer," they will continue to select the category and the point value.
- If the team incorrectly formed a "question" for the given "answer," the moderator will indicate that it is an incorrect question and give the other team the opportunity to form a question.
- If the second team is able to correctly form a "question" for the given "answer," their team will receive the points and take control of the game board.
- If the second team is unable to correctly form a "question" for the given "answer," the moderator will direct the computer operator to show the correct "question" and the control of the board will remain with the first team.
- The play continues until all the categories and point values have been selected.
- The moderator will announce the winner from the cumulative score sheet.

You can change these directions and "rules" in any way that works for your situation. It is important, however, to establish the rules ahead of time. The moderator also has the opportunity to discuss any of the "answers" and "questions" at the conclusion of each response. If, for example, neither team is able to form a correct question, the moderator may use this as an opportunity to talk about the "answer" and "question."

MODIFICATION OF THE CISM CHALLENGE GAME

To modify this game with your own questions and answers, follow these directions:

- Go to the main PowerPoint screen with the smaller screen on the right hand side showing the content of the selected slide and the slide text going down the left side of the screen.
- The answers begin with slide #5, followed on slide #6 with the correct answer. To change any or all of the questions, just overtype the existing text. Remember, the answer slide is always followed by the question slide.
- You can also edit the questions and answers at the small slide screen on the right hand side.
- Go to slide #5 (either by scrolling down on the slide bar to the right of the slide screen or by selecting the slide icon in the left-hand screen) and you see the text "THIS MAN FORMALIZED THE ICISF MODEL."
- Highlight this text and type whatever answer you want. Move to the next slide where you find the question, "WHO IS DR. JEFFREY T. MITCHELL?" and again highlight the text and modify the question.

It is strongly recommended that you save your modification to a floppy disk.

FRIENDLY FRACAS GAME

INSTRUCTIONS FOR LOADING AND OPERATING

- Open and print the file **FriendlyFracasQ&A.pdf** on the CD-ROM which contains the questions and answers for the game. If a computer operator is assisting the moderator, it will be easier to have two printed copies of this document.
- Open or run PowerPoint on your computer and select the file **FriendlyFracas.PPT** which is also on the CD-ROM.
- View the game in slide show mode by selecting the "slide show" icon in the lower left tool bar (or by pressing the F5 function key) and you will get the title screen.
- Depress the space bar one time and the game board screen will appear (the question, three white boxes, and eight buttons).
- After the moderator reads the question and the first person who raises his/her hand gives an answer, the computer operator will determine if that answer appears on the board by referring to the "Q&A" document.
- There are eight buttons at the bottom of the game board (see diagram in "Q&A" document). Button #1 displays the first correct answer, button #2 displays the second correct answer, button #3 displays the third correct answer. Button #4 displays answers 1 and 2, button #5 displays answers 1 and 3, and button #6 displays answers 2 and 3. Button #7 displays all the correct answers and button #8 takes you to the next question.
- After the first correct answer is given, the computer operator will select the appropriate button according to the Q&A sheet and that answer with the number of people responding to it will appear on the screen. To return to the game board screen, the computer operator will then click on the single button in the lower right-hand corner of the screen.
- After the second correct answer is given, the computer operator will click one of the buttons in the second group which will show the number of people responding. To return to the game board screen, the computer operator will then click the single button in the lower right-hand corner of the screen.
- When all three correct answers are given, the computer operator will click on button #7 that will display all three correct answers and the number of people responding with that answer are displayed on the screen.
- When all three correct answers are displayed on the game board, the computer operator will click on button #8 to move the game to the next question.

GROUP INSTRUCTIONS

- Project the first slide on the computer screen (FRIENDLY FRACAS and two hands shaking).
- Select two teams of five players (or any number you wish) to play the game.
- Arrange the players so that they can all see the computer screen or the projection screen.
- Select three judges to determine who raises his/her hand first when the answer is shown on the screen. All participants agree to accept the ruling of the majority of the judges on who raised his/her hand first. If you are fortunate enough to have game paddles that identify who signaled first, second, and third, then you won't need to appoint judges.
- Project the second slide on the screen by depressing the space bar once. This screen will have the question across the top, three white boxes, and eight round buttons at the bottom of the screen.
- The moderator will read the first question and the first person from either team who raises his/her hand will be allowed to answer the question. If the answer is one of the three answers provided by the survey, the person operating the computer will display the answer and point value. (Please note this is different from the popular game show in which each team is able to answer and the highest one chooses to play or pass.)
- The computer operator will then return the screen back to the main screen.
- The play will continue with the team answering with the highest score until they either correctly name all three responses or make two errors.
- If the first team makes two errors, the other team will have the opportunity to "steal" by giving an answer that has not already been selected.
- If the second team is able to give a correct answer, they will take all the points on the board. If the second team is unable to give another correct answer, the first team will keep any points they have accumulated.

You can change these directions and "rules" in any way that works for your situation. It is important, however, to establish the rules ahead of time. The moderator also has the opportunity to discuss any of the survey questions or responses.

MODIFICATION OF THE FRIENDLY FRACAS GAME

If you choose to modify this game, you should be aware of how hyperlinks work in PowerPoint. All of the hyperlinks will need to be changed if you add or delete any slides. If you only change the wording on the slides, the game will function properly.

- Go to the main PowerPoint screen with the smaller screen on the right-hand side showing the content of the selected slide and the slide text going down the left side of the screen.
- Change any answer by over-writing **each** of the four times the answer and point value appears.
- If you notice that the survey answer or point value doesn't line up properly, go to the smaller screen on the right hand side and add spaces or delete spaces until they line up properly.

It is strongly recommended that you save your modification to a floppy disk.

QUESTION ME THIS GAME

INSTRUCTIONS FOR LOADING AND OPERATING

- Open or run PowerPoint on your computer.
- Select the file QUESTION ME THIS.PPT on the CD ROM included with this book.
- Select the slide show icon in the lower left tool bar (icon of a screen) and you will get the title screen full size.
- To advance to the next slide press the space bar. Each time you press the space bar, the next slide will appear which has the question and answer.

The moderator should review all the "answers" and "questions" prior to playing the game. This game is meant to reinforce teaching that has already taken place. The examples presented here may contain information that you have not already taught. You can either present this information or modify the "answers" and "questions" to material with which your participants are familiar.

The computer operator should practice several times with the program before actually playing the game so that he/she is familiar with how to operate it. It is also a good idea to have a printed copy of all the slides with the computer operator. To print a copy of the slides while the program is loaded, select print from the File Option. In the lower left hand corner there is a box that is entitled "Print What." Select one of the options and then select how you want it printed by checking the appropriate box.

GROUP INSTRUCTIONS

- Project the first slide on the computer screen (QUESTION ME THIS).
- Select two teams of three players (or any number you wish) to play the game.
- Arrange them so that they can all see the computer screen or the projection screen.
- Select three judges to determine who raises his/her hand first when the answer is shown on the screen. All participants agree to accept the ruling of the majority of the judges on who raised his/her hand first. If you are fortunate enough to have game paddles that identify who signaled first, second, and third, then you won't need to appoint judges.
- Project the second and third slides, which are informational slides, on the screen by depressing the space bar.
- Project the next slide by depressing the space bar. An "answer" will appear.
- The moderator will call on the first person identified by the judges to provide an appropriate question.
- At the direction from the moderator, depress the space bar again and the "question" will be displayed on the screen with the question.

- One of the judges will mark 10 points for the team on a cumulative score sheet which is large enough for everyone to see.
- If the team incorrectly formed a "question" for the given "answer," the moderator will indicate that it is an incorrect question and instruct the judge/scorekeeper to deduct 10 points from the team on a cumulative score sheet which is large enough for everyone to see.
- When the moderator calls for the next "answer," the computer operator will depress the space bar again.
- The play continues until all "answers" and "questions" have been completed.
- Near the end of the game, players have the opportunity to wager points they have earned against some additional questions.
- The moderator will announce the winner from the cumulative score sheet.

You can change these directions and "rules" in any way that works for your situation. It is important, however, to establish the rules ahead of time. The moderator also has the opportunity to discuss any of the "answers" and "questions" at the conclusion of each response. If, for example, neither team is able to form a correct question, the moderator may use this as an opportunity to talk about the "answer" and "question."

MODIFICATION OF THE QUESTION ME THIS GAME

To modify this game with your own questions and answers, follow these directions:

- Go to the main PowerPoint screen with the smaller screen on the right hand side showing the content of the selected slide and the slide text going down the left side of the screen.
- The answers begin with slide #4 with the "answer" first and then the "question." To change any or all of the questions/answers, just overtype the existing text.
- You can also edit the questions and answers at the small slide screen on the right hand side.

It is strongly recommended that you save your modification to a floppy disk.

WHO WANTS TO BE A DEBRIEFER?

INSTRUCTIONS FOR LOADING AND OPERATING

- Open or run PowerPoint on your computer.
- Select the file WHO WANTS TO BE A DEBRIEFER?.PPT on the CD ROM included with this book.
- Select the slide show icon in the lower left tool bar (icon of a screen) and you will get the title screen full size.
- To advance to the next slide press the space bar. Each time you press the space bar, the next slide will appear which has the question and answer.

The moderator should review all the "questions" and "multiple choice answers" prior to playing the game. It is meant to reinforce teaching that has already taken place. The examples presented here may contain information that you have not already taught. You can either present this information or modify the "questions" and "multiple choice answers" to material with which your participants are familiar.

The computer operator should practice several times with the program before actually playing the game so that he/she is familiar with how to operate it. It is also a good idea to have a printed copy of all the slides with the computer operator. To print a copy of the slides while the program is loaded, select print from the File Option. In the lower left hand corner there is a box that is entitled "Print What." Select one of the options and then select how you want it printed by checking the appropriate box.

GROUP INSTRUCTIONS

- Project the first slide on the computer screen (WHO WANTS TO BE A DEBRIEFER?).
- Select one person to play the game. The player gets to pick three people to be his consultants.
- Arrange them so that he/she can see the computer screen or the projection screen.
- The first question is on the next slide. When the computer operator depresses the space bar, the questions and four possible answers will appear.
- The contestant (with consultation, if he/she wishes) will select the best answer from the choices provided.
- At the direction from the moderator, depress the space bar again and the correct answer will be displayed on the screen.
- One of the judges will mark 10 points for the correct answer.
- If the contestant incorrectly answers the question, the moderator will indicate that it is an incorrect answer and instruct the judge/scorekeeper to deduct 10 points from his/her cumulative score.

- When the moderator calls for the next question, the computer operator will depress the space bar again.
- When the contestant has answered his/her 10 questions, another contestant will be selected.
- The play continues until all "questions" and "answers" have been completed.
- The moderator will announce the winner from the cumulative score sheet.

You can change these directions and "rules" in any way that works for your situation. It is important, however, to establish the rules ahead of time. The moderator also has the opportunity to discuss any of the "questions" and "answers" at the conclusion of each response. If, for example, neither team is able to form a correct question, the moderator may use this as an opportunity to talk about the "question" and "answer."

MODIFICATION OF THE WHO WANTS TO BE A DEBRIEFER GAME

To modify this game with your own questions and answers, follow these directions:

- Go to the main PowerPoint screen with the smaller screen on the right hand side showing the content of the selected slide and the slide text going down the left side of the screen.
- The questions/answers begin with slide number 2. To change any or all of the questions/ answers, just overtype the existing text.
- You can also edit the questions and answers at the small slide screen on the right hand side.

It is strongly recommended that you save your modification to a floppy disk.

Appendix 1

MODEL FOR DEBRIEFING

Introductory Phase

All Groups

- Introduce the team members.
- This is not a critique.
- You do not have to talk, but what you say may help someone else.
- Ask participants to respect the privacy of others.
- No breaks are planned.
- Do not say anything that would incriminate you.
- No pagers or cell phone calls.
- This group is for _________. Look around the room. Is anyone here who should not be?
- Feel free to ask questions.

EMS Personnel

- No one has rank here.
- This defusing/debriefing is **not** part of any investigating agency.
- Turn off radios and pagers (you are off-duty).

Describe what is going to occur. There will be three questions to which each participant is asked to respond. Ask each participant in the group to give his/her name the first time around.

Fact Phase

Community

- Who are you?
- What was your relationship to the victim?
- Where were you at the time of the incident?
- What happened?

EMS Personnel

- Give your name and describe what you did at the scene?
- What happened?
- What happened from your point of view?

Thought Phase

Community

- What thought has been stuck in your head since the event?

EMS Personnel

- Share your first thought when you came off "auto-pilot."
- What were your first thoughts during the event?

Reaction Phase

Community

- What were some of your immediate reactions?
- What reactions are you having now?
- What was the **worst** thing about the event for you?
- If you could change one thing (but still not change the outcome), what would that be?

EMS Personnel

- Share what you saw as the worst part of the incident?
- What was the **worst** thing about the event?
- If you could change one thing (but still not change the outcome), what would that be?

Symptom Phase

All Groups

- What have you noticed about yourself that is different since the event?
- Please share information about any reactions you have experienced or are experiencing:
  — Physical reactions
  — Emotional reactions
  — Cognitive reactions
  — Behavioral reactions
- Is your experience today the same as it was at the scene or the following day?

Teaching Phase

Community and EMS

- Reassure the participants that these are normal reactions to the situation—normal reactions of a **normal** individual to an **abnormal** event.
- You had no control over what happened. You do have some control over how you cope with it.
- When appropriate, the following sentence may be helpful, "I could have, I should have, if only I had of. Oh my God, it is all my fault."
- Discuss handouts.
- Discuss coping strategies.

Re-Entry Phase

Community and EMS

- Wrap up any loose ends, indicate sources of additional assistance, and encourage participants to be supportive of each other through the next few days.
- Indicate that while this defusing/debriefing begins the healing process, the participants may continue to experience reactions for the next few days or weeks. Have each person state one thing they are going to do to take care of themselves.
- Any "plan of action" needed?
- Ask if there is anything any of the participants would like to say that they were not given the opportunity say.
- Remind the participants about confidentiality.

DEBRIEFING THE DEBRIEFERS

Ask each defuser/debriefer the following questions:

- In general, how do you think the defusing/debriefing went?
- Is there anything you said that you wish now that you had not said?
- Is there anything that you did not say that you wish that you had said?
- What inappropriate thing, if anything, did you do during the defusing/debriefing?
- Is there anything that the coordinator could have done prior to the defusing/debriefing that would have helped you?
- What are you going to do for **yourself** when you go home?

Appendix 2

QUESTIONS COORDINATORS ASK

About the Incident:

- What happened?
- Why do you think that this is a critical incident?
- Are other departments or agencies involved?
- Exactly when and where did it happen:
- Is the event really over?
- Who was involved?
- Is there continuing rescue or recovery ongoing?
- How many individuals were involved?
- What are the employees saying about the event?

Suddenness:

- Was timing or location especially unexpected?
- Was home or workplace invaded?
- Was the impact disorienting?

Severity:

- Were there multiple victims?
- Is this affecting families or other less involved employees, customers, bystanders?
- Was there exposure to gruesome sensory factors (sights, sounds, smells, etc.)?
- Is this affecting the agency's ability to operate?
- Were there any child victims involved?
- Were there any coworkers involved?
- Were any of the victims known to members of the group?
- Were any individuals in fear of their own death?

Proximity:

- Was there any physical contact with the victim (blood, etc.)?
- Were there any witnesses to death?
- Was there any thought that "this could have been any of us"?

Other Complicating Factors:

- Was there a crime involved?
- Is the perpetrator at large?
- Is age or developmental level a factor?
- Is there any media exposure?
- Is there any direct criticism from the media?
- Are languages or cultural differences a factor?

Timing and Logistics:

- Is timing of a funeral or other service an issue in when the response is held?
- Is the agency keeping participants “on the clock”?
- Should there be some interventions immediately?
- Should there be some interventions later?
- Where should the response be held?
- If multiple agencies are involved, can they be mixed?
- Has the invitation for services been approved by the administration?
- When can all participants be off-call?
- Has the host agency agreed to ground rules?

About the Group:

- Should supervisors be in the response? Involved in the event? Generally trusted?
- Does this group have multiple or cumulative issues?
- Has any group member had recent or similar losses?
- Is there any blaming going on? If yes, who and how prevalent?
- Has the group had previous CISM services and what was their reaction to the previous intervention?
- Is there any internal investigation under way?
- Is there a threat to anyone’s job?
- Is sub-grouping a factor (labor vs. management, etc.)?
- What is the general level of trust among this group?
- Are there any legal concerns?
- Were any mistakes made (honest, procedural errors, etc.)?

Appendix 3

MEMORANDUM OF UNDERSTANDING FOR TEAM MEMBERSHIP

I hereby agree to serve as a volunteer of the ___________ CISM team. As a member, I agree to the following expectations:

1. To participate in CISM training programs to maintain my CISM skills.
2. To participate in scheduled team meetings on a regular basis.
3. To participate in team CISM responses as called upon, when possible.
4. To maintain strict confidentiality regarding any and all CISM activities and not to divulge any information regarding incidents, locations, personnel involved, or other aspects of the CISM meetings, and then not relating names or specifics.
5. To complete all required reports and submit these to the on-call coordinator within one week of the activity.

I further agree to support the mission and best interests of the __________ CISM team and to promote its growth and positive reputation within the community and within the CISM network.

I shall not misuse my membership on this team for my own personal gain or agenda, or make claims about my membership that might hurt the team in any fashion.

I fully understand that any breach of confidentiality regarding any of the CISM activities that I participate in, or become knowledgeable about, and/or any performance of activities deemed to be in a direct conflict of interest with the team, may result in immediate removal from the team.

Signature: ___________________________________

Date: _______________________________________

Appendix 4

CRITICAL INCIDENT SERVICE REQUEST

1. INITIAL CONTACT

Received from: ______________________ Date: ______________

Contact person: ______________________________________

Home phone: ____________________ Work phone: ______________

Agency name: ____

Address: ____

Chief administrator: ___________________________________

Is this person aware of the request? θ Yes θ No

Telephone number, if different: ____________________________

2. INCIDENT

Nature of incident: _____________________________________

____

____

Date/time of incident: ___________________________________

Location: ____

Agencies involved: ______________________________________

Urgency of request: θ Immediate θ Within 24 hours θ Within 72 hours

3. IN-HOUSE CISM RESPONSE UNDER WAY? θ Yes θ No

Contact person: ______________________ Phone: ______________

4. STATE CISM RESPONSE UNDER WAY? θ Yes θ No

Contact person: ______________________ Phone: ______________

5. **ACTION TAKEN:**

Request approved / team activated: θ Yes θ No

Names of the event team: ______________________________

____

Rendezvous point: ______________________________

Directions: ______________________________

____

Time: ______________________________

Date and time of debriefing: ______________________________

Location of debriefing: ______________________________

Directions to location: ______________________________

____

Debriefing for (specify populations): ______________________________

Size of group expected: ______________________________

Request denied: ______________________________

Reason: ______________________________

____

Services offered: ______________________________

Additional information: ______________________________

____

____

____

____

____

____

6. **RECORDER'S NAME:** ______________________________

Appendix 5

INTERVENTION REPORTING FORM

Team name: ______________________________ County: ________________________

Date of intervention: ____ /____ /____

Day of the week: Sun M T W Th F Sat

Type of agency(ies) / group served: ____

Number of participants: ____________________________

Number of team members: ____________________________

Intervention (see "A" below): ________________________

Community / EMS? ______________________________

Event involved (see "B" below): ______________________

A. INTERVENTIONS

a. Pre-crisis preparation
b. Demobilization
c. Staff consultation
d. Crisis management briefing (CMB)
e. Defusing
f. Critical incident stress debriefing
g. Individual crisis intervention
h. Pastoral crisis
i. Family CISM
j. Organizational consultation
k. Follow-ups
l. Referral

B. EVENTS

a. Accident
b. Armed robbery
c. Business / factory downsizing
d. Disaster / multiple deaths
e. Fire death
f. School crisis
g. Infant / child injury / death
h. Knowing the victim
i. Line of duty / serious injury or death
j. School crisis
k. School violence
l. Sudden death
m. Suicide
n. Workplace accident
o. Workplace violence
p. Act of terrorism
q. Other (explain ____________)

Appendix 6

INCIDENT COORDINATOR'S ROSTER

RESPONSES FOR THE YEAR 20___

DATE	TYPE	AGENCY(IES)	PARTICIPANTS	DEBRIEFERS

Appendix 7

COORDINATOR'S FOLLOW-UP / OUTCOME QUESTIONS

Remember, a good CISM response rarely consists of a single intervention. Think follow-up.

After the team has completed an intervention, the coordinator should make contact with the administration of the organization served to find out how the team's efforts were perceived and to assess need for further services.

A few specific goals of this contact are:

- To solicit feedback on satisfaction
- To learn how to improve procedures
- To continue triage or identification of individuals who may require further assistance
- To assess need for further interventions, of any type

The following questions are suggestions to help meet the above goals:

- Can you give me a general reaction about the efforts of our team?
- Is there any specific feedback the team should hear?
- Have you noticed any differences in the way your employees are talking to each other since our response?
- Are there any specific improvements in employee functioning, attendance, or morale?
- Do you still have employees who are unable to work because of the incident?
- Would anyone like a one-on-one follow-up conversation?
- Are employees still expressing concern about how this event continues to affect members of their family?
- Is the event causing ongoing public relations problems in the community your agency serves (i.e., need for CMB)?
- Are there aspects which might respond better to pastoral crisis intervention?
- Would you please remember to collect the "Debriefing Feedback Forms" which we distributed and drop them in the mail to us?
- Would you like to have a visit from one of our team coordinators to discuss the services we offer?

Appendix 8

DEBRIEFING FEEDBACK FORM

Instructions: *Please allow at least 24 hours to pass before you fill out this form. Your feedback is important to us. It is a vital piece of information used when evaluating our program.*

1. The month before the traumatic event, I was feeling:
   Bad .... 1 .... 2 .... 3 .... 4 .... 5 .... Good

2. After the traumatic event, I was feeling:
   Upset .... 1 .... 2 .... 3 .... 4 .... 5 .... Calm

3. I found the debriefing to be:
   Harmful .... 1 .... 2 .... 3 .... 4 .... 5 .... Helpful

4. How clear were the group leaders in presenting introductions, ground rules and reasoning behind the debriefings?
   Confusing .... 1 .... 2 .... 3 .... 4 .... 5 .... Clear

5. How helpful was it to talk about your reactions:?
   Harmful .... 1 .... 2 .... 3 .... 4 .... 5 .... Helpful

6. How helpful was it to listen to the reactions of other group members?
   Harmful .... 1 .... 2 .... 3 .... 4 .... 5 .... Helpful

7. How helpful was it to hear about the physical reactions of the other group members?
   Harmful .... 1 .... 2 .... 3 .... 4 .... 5 .... Helpful

8. How helpful was it to talk about how the traumatic event affected your thinking?
   Harmful .... 1 .... 2 .... 3 .... 4 .... 5 .... Helpful

9. How helpful was it to hear about how the traumatic event affected the thinking of other group members?
   Harmful .... 1 .... 2 .... 3 .... 4 .... 5 .... Helpful

10. How helpful were the handouts about common stress reactions and methods to care for yourself?
    Harmful .... 1 .... 2 .... 3 .... 4 .... 5 .... Helpful

11. How helpful were the group leaders in encouraging discussion?
    Harmful .... 1 .... 2 .... 3 .... 4 .... 5 .... Helpful

12. Comments? (Please use the back side of this form)

Adapted from material from Gryphon Place, Kalamazoo, Michigan. Used with permission.

Appendix 9

OBSERVER'S FEEDBACK FORM FOR ONE-ON-ONES

How did the speaker perform in the following areas?

1. Use of silence

2. Use of body language/posture that was conducive to communication

3. Appropriate choice of verbal language

4. Use of restatement

5. Use of emotional reflection

6. Use of paraphrasing

7. Use of summary statements

8. Use of the appropriate structured ICISF model (3-step, 5-step, or 7-step)

9. Did the conversation have a natural flow?

10. What was the most helpful statement made?

11. What would have been more helpful?

Adapted from G. Everly and J. Mitchell (1998) *Assisting Individuals in Crisis: A Workbook*, Chevron Publishing. Used with permission.

Appendix 10

CISD OBSERVATION FORM

As you observe the small group role play, use this format to assist in giving feedback to the debriefing team.

INTRODUCTION:

Appropriate introductions?
Purpose clearly stated?
Ground rules clearly delineated?
Strengths?
Suggestions for change?

FACT:

Effective transition?
Purpose clearly stated?
Limited comments to facts of event?
Strengths?
Suggestions for change?

THOUGHT:

Effective transition?
Thoughts clarified?
Strengths?
Suggestions for change?

REACTION:

Effective transition?
Provided for validation of experience?
Encouraged the group to be supportive?
Facilitated without dominating discussion?
Strengths?
Suggestions for change?

SYMPTOM:

Effective transition?
Symptoms normalized?
Strengths?
Suggestions for change?

Adapted from *Critical Incident Stress Management: Advanced Group Crisis Interventions / A Workbook:* Chevron Publishing. Used with permission.

TEACHING:

Effective transition?
Practical teaching based upon issues presented by the group?
Group material used?
Strengths?
Suggestions for change?

RE-ENTRY:

Effective summarization?
Effective closure?
Strengths?
Suggestions for change?

OVERALL REVIEW OF EXPERIENCE:

Comment on the team using each other.

Comment on the timing of moving the group along and transitioning between phases (did it "feel" right?).

It is a good idea to end with a positive. What was one of the best things you saw this team do?

Appendix 11

SUGGESTED READING

These are some of the books that are helpful for a coordinator, clinical director, or educational facilitator to have available. There is a significant body of work on more specialized areas of crisis response, workplace violence, and responding to schools. These can be found by obtaining a complete list from Chevron Publishing Corporation at their website ***www.chevronpublishing.com****.*

Mitchell, J.T. and Everly, G.S., Jr. (2001). ***Critical Incident Stress Debriefing: An Operations Manual for CISD, Defusing and Other Group Crisis Intervention Services. 3rd Edition.***, Ellicott City, MD: Chevron Publishing Corporation.

Everly, G.S. and Mitchell, J.T. (1999) ***Critical Incident Stress Management: A New Era and Standard of Care In Crisis Intervention, 2nd Edition.*** Ellicott City, MD: Chevron Publishing Corporation.

Mitchell, J.T. and Everly, G.S., Jr. (1994). ***Human Elements Training For Emergency Services, Public Safety and Disaster Personnel: An Instructional Guide to Teaching Debriefing, Crisis Intervention And Stress Management Porgrams***. Ellicott City, MD: Chevron Publishing Corporation.

Mitchell, J.T. and Resnick, H.L.P. (1986). ***Emergency Response To Crisis***. Ellicott City, MD: Chevron Publishing Corporation.

Robinson, R. and Murdock, P. (1998). ***Guidelines for Establishing and Maintaining Peer Support Programs in Emergency Services, 2nd Edition***. Ellicott City, MD: Chevron Publishing Corporation.

Flannery, R. B. Jr., (1998). ***The Assaulted Staff Action Program: Coping with the Psychological Aftermath of Violence.*** Ellicott City, MD: Chevron Publishing Corporation.

Flannery, R. B. Jr., (1994). ***Becoming Stress Resistant – Through the Project SMART Program.*** Ellicott City, MD: Chevron Publishing Corporation.

Johnson, K. (2000). ***School Crisis Management.*** Ellicott City, MD: Chevron Publishing Corporation.

Schoenfeld, M. (1993) ***School Crisis Response Teams: Lessening the Aftermath***; Ellicott City, MD: Chevron Publishing Corporation.

Casey, D. and Leger, E. (1996). ***Rural Emergency Response: A Guide to Coping with Stressors in Rural Emergency Services Delivery***. Ellicott City, MD: Chevron Publishing Corporation.